Accidentally OVER- WEIGHT

Other books by Dr. Libby :

Exhausted to Energized (2015)

The Calorie Fallacy (2014)

Sweet Food Story (2014)

Beauty From the Inside Out (2013)

Real Food Kitchen (2013)

Real Food Chef (2012)

Rushing Woman's Syndrome (2011)

(All titles published by Little Green Frog Publishing Ltd.)

Accidentally OVER-WEIGHT

The 9 Elements That Will Help
You Solve Your Weight-Loss Puzzle

Dr. Libby Weaver

HAY HOUSE

Carlsbad, California • New York City • London • Sydney
Johannesburg • Vancouver • Hong Kong • New Delhi

Published and distributed in the United States by: Hay House, Inc.: www .hayhouse.com® • **Published and distributed in Australia by:** Hay House Australia Pty. Ltd.: www.hayhouse.com.au • **Published and distributed in the United Kingdom by:** Hay House UK, Ltd.: www.hayhouse.co.uk • **Published and distributed in the Republic of South Africa by:** Hay House SA (Pty), Ltd.: www.hayhouse.co.za • **Distributed in Canada by:** Raincoast Books: www.raincoast.com • **Published in India by:** Hay House Publishers India: www.hayhouse.co.in

Cover and interior design: Leanne Siu Anastasi • Interior images: p. 3 iStock; all other images © Dr. Libby Weaver

Library of Congress Control Number: 2015953600

Tradepaper ISBN: 978-1-4019-5023-1

10 9 8 7 6 5 4 3 2 1
1st edition, March 2016

Printed in the United States of America

SUSTAINABLE
FORESTRY
INITIATIVE
Certified Chain of Custody
Promoting Sustainable Forestry
www.sfiprogram.org
SFI-01268
SFI label applies to the text stock

For Christopher,
with spectacular gratitude.

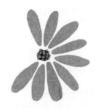

Contents

Acknowledgments

To the amazing Chris Weaver. Thank you for your passion, your humor, your eyes, your arms, your immense generosity and opening me to a new phase of learning and discovery. Thank you for being a guiding light for me and helping me take my messages to the world. You surprise and delight me and I adore you.

To my dear Mum and Dad. Thank you for the way you raised me and for loving me unconditionally. I am who I am mostly because of you both and I wouldn't be doing this work without the gifts of my delightful childhood. Mum, thank you for being the kindest lady on the planet and my best friend. Thank you Dad for being the wonderful provider and friend that you have always been to me, and for having chickens and parsley in the backyard.

John Aiken, aka J. Dizzle, thank you for sharing the "Accidentally" name with me. John is a psychologist who has written a wonderful book called *Accidentally Single*. Thanks for sharing and for encouraging me to fly above the radar.

Thank you to a very special place on this Earth called Gwinganna Lifestyle Retreat (Queensland, Australia) for her nurturing of me. The land and the passionate, life-loving people that make up this amazing place will always have a sense of home for me. I am eternally grateful to the process a stay at Gwinganna offers her guests, for it is through this process that I first caught a glimpse of the biochemistry and the psychology of what I now call *Accidentally Overweight*. Big love to Sharon and Karl.

Thank you to Petrea for her belief in me, and the way she encouraged me to get this out there and for being such fun. You rock!

Thank you to my precious Miss Bliss (hi Bella!) for her magical heart and her unconditional love for me. Thank you! I love you. Thanks to Leisel and Ruby Red Rose for the cutest voicemails ever during the biggest work (mission) year of my life so far and to all of my friends' patience while I hibernated and wrote this beloved book and spent no time on the phone.

Thanks will always go to Professor Tim Roberts and Associate Professor Hugh Dunstan for their passion for bugs (gut and infective), steroid hormones, biochemistry, immunology, and microbiology, and the inspiration they offered before and during my PhD to explore the whys behind numerous health conditions. And to Dr. Merv Garrett for smashing my brain wide open back in 1997 and being the original pioneer; you changed the course of my life and I am forever grateful to you.

Thank you to Tony and Sage Robbins for their gifts of insight into the tremendous heart of real human psychology. Tony you are a genius and Sage your feminine essence is a gift to the world. Massive thanks and recognition to Deborah Battersby for her contribution to the world, most recently in the form of Em-Matrix, and for her deep caring. Thank you to Louise Hay for her pioneering work into the metaphysical basis of health conditions. There are times when the lessons I have learned from all of these people have allowed a client to open to what was really at the heart of their health challenge. As I love to say, "It is never about the food. And yet it is about the food for that is some people's doorway to their own magnificence."

Thank you to the children with autism who, through my work with them and their families, gave me an insight into far more than just gut function and poo! Like canaries in the mines, these children are a gift offering us also a warning that we cannot continue living in the way that we are. Our world is too toxic for them. And the *Accidentally Overweight* are but just one more sign of this.

To everyone who knows somewhere inside of them that it is not about the food, I hope you are reminded throughout these pages of what you already know.

• • • • • • • • • • • • •

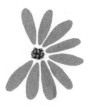

Guidelines for Getting the Most Out of This Book

Please read this whole book. Do not just go to the solutions section at the end of each puzzle piece, or chapter, because you won't understand *why* specific changes are being recommended. You'll also find solutions are offered the whole way through each and every chapter, and you may miss these if you don't read everything. There is also a reason for the order of the chapters.

Information is expanded upon as the book continues and we move from the physical—body-fat accumulation—through to the emotional, and along the way you'll see how they are all linked. Nothing stands alone in our chemistry. Also, to truly get the immense benefits from the final piece of the puzzle, emotions, you need to know the stories that led up to this chapter, which you'll find presented throughout the book. So please read it from cover to cover and soak it up.

Do not go straight to the emotions chapter, even if you believe that this is the only part you don't yet understand. *Accidentally Overweight* was written as a sequence, so that the information and experiences unfold as you read it from the first page through to the last. Once you have read it all, by all means return to any place you like.

You may notice that throughout the book I often write "we," and this is because I am used to working as a team with my clients. Even though I am not physically with you as you read this book, I want you to feel like I'm someone who understands. The details of people's lives are very different, yet the patterns of responses driving human behavior are often very similar.

There are sections of *Accidentally Overweight* that may seem more geared to a female audience. But the messages in the book are just as relevant to men, even if in certain sections men are simply given the opportunity to understand the women in their lives better. This is particularly true of Puzzle Piece 3, Sex Hormones.

You will see throughout the book that each chapter contains a checklist to help you identify whether a particular puzzle piece might be relevant to you. It is important to note that not all of these signs need to be present for the puzzle piece to be playing a role in the heath picture of an individual. Reading each chapter of this book is designed to help you decipher whether a particular puzzle piece is likely to be part of your health picture. If a chapter resonates strongly, that puzzle piece likely needs attention. If not, then simply learn from the information.

Also, the signs and symptoms listed for each puzzle piece are not finite. Please note, too, that some of the signs and symptoms can be representative of other heath conditions or diseases, and that these checklists infer that more sinister causes have been ruled out by a medical professional.

As I came to evolve my concept of *Accidentally Overweight* more deeply, what began as a random scribble on the page grew into a pie chart, which I'd ask clients to complete so we could establish the areas where they needed support.

Although today I use the image of a puzzle to depict the concept of *Accidentally Overweight*, this simply serves to illustrate that often numerous pieces have to come together for an individual to reach their weight-loss and health goals.

For you to get the most out of this book, I am going to encourage you to begin where I begin with all of my clients—with the pie chart. As you come to the end of each chapter, I'd like you to score yourself for that particular area, not based on a rating of "good" or "bad" but on a scale of one to ten. Ten indicates that this piece of your chart needs absolutely no support or attention—you have that section sorted—while a score of one indicates that you have identified that this particular area needs a significant amount of support and attention. Once you have scored yourself for each puzzle piece, return to the pie chart, mark your scores in each area, and then color in your wheel. The more white space, the more support you need to focus on that area. Most people notice that if their chart were actually a wheel, it wouldn't be able to turn. It would get stuck in one or more areas.

Identifying the areas where you need support allows you to focus on the information and solutions most relevant to your health. After you have implemented some or all of the strategies suggested in the section/s relevant to you for four-week periods, you can return to your chart and use a different colored marker to identify your new scores. Your goal is not necessarily to get to ten in all areas. Identify the roadblocks to your fat burning and aim to have more colored areas in your chart. Get your scores (your biochemistry) to a point where your weight-loss wheel begins to turn again, generating the health outcomes you desire.

> *"If the answers to what you are searching for were in the places you had already been looking, don't you think you would have found them by now?"*
>
> Anonymous

It is time to look at food, health, and your body in a brand new way.

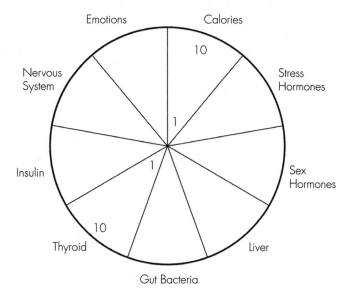

Figure 1: Your Accidently Overweight Puzzle

A Little Background...

Before beginning, I want to reflect on human history so you can begin to appreciate truly just how miraculous our bodies are and also some powerful reasons why human health has shifted so significantly in the past 30 or so years.

I'm not talking about human evolution in the sense of biblical "creation" versus Darwinian "evolution." Instead, let this be a brief exploration of the major milestones in the evolution of the human body and biochemistry.

Human beings have been on Earth for between 150,000 and 200,000 years. We have evolved slowly and steadily over time, and, as nomads, lived off the land that surrounded us as we moved. We were hunters and gatherers and the seasons, the climate, and the weather conditions predominantly influenced our food choices. Humans ate fresh food precisely the way it came from nature. Our diet was based primarily on plants, and other more concentrated foods were added when the opportunity arose from hunting and gathering.

Approximately 7,500 to 10,000 years ago, humans started to stay in one place for longer periods of time, and basic agricultural practices were established. This was the first time we grew crops and the first time in human history that we consumed the milk of other animals. This was also the first time that repetition became significant in the human diet, as a result of not having to chase our food down, and also having a supply of crops in the field. Our patterns of eating, however, were still based on nature's rhythms, and our produce was seasonal and at the mercy of floods and droughts.

While change continued at a very gradual, steady pace, the chemistry developments in our body could keep up. The next most significant change to our lifestyles came during the 19th century, as a result of the Industrial Revolution. Processes were mechanized, and people started to move in big numbers from the country to the cities. There was an enormous reliance on agriculture for food production as population numbers continued to grow, and a day's work now required less movement as people came off the land and worked in the newly developed factories.

Propel forward to today. I believe that when historians review our time on the planet, they will identify the past two decades—which have included the invention of cell phones and the birth of the Internet—as the most rapid period of change in human history. We now eat out of packets, which contain numbers (including additives and preservatives) rather than food-based ingredients, and live our lives in front of screens. We don't have to climb stairs, as there are elevators, escalators, and moving walkways. We don't even have to go to the store to buy our food, let alone go into the fields and harvest it or chase it with a spear. We can order it online and have someone deliver it.

There is no judgment here. Just a tip-of-the-iceberg observation of how quickly and significantly the world in which we live has changed. We are guinea pigs in so many areas. Never before has a group of people been exposed to pesticides for their entire lives. Never before have there been artificial sweeteners, colors, and preservatives in our food for the entirety of our lifetimes. I am crossing every finger and toe and even my eyes in the hope that they are safe. My instinct tells me they are not.

We have also witnessed a rapid expansion of the human frame and waistline. As hygiene practices have improved, along with nutrition generally, we have literally grown to new heights. Unfortunately, our waistlines have grown, too, which is both a sign and a consequence of our times.

At a cellular level, we have basically the same human body as our ancestors. Every generation evolves ever so slightly to be better equipped to inhabit its environment. This rate of evolution, however, is nothing compared to the change of pace in the world. Our conscious minds may have developed to keep up with the times, so that we are able to email while we talk on our cell phone at the same time as we remember that we must pick up the children from school, but biochemically we are much the same as we were 150,000 years ago. Still the same, too, is our subconscious mind, which is infinitely more powerful than our conscious mind. The subconscious mind makes our heart beat and our hair grow. It knows how to heal a cut without you having to tell it to do so. Don't you think that is amazing? I do not believe that our nervous systems, which enormously affect every cell of our bodies, every hormonal system, every organ, every aspect of fat burning, have been able to keep up with the rate of change that this time in human history demands of us.

Between our laptops and wireless modems, our cell phones and email systems, we are asking our bodies to go places they have never ever been before. Never have we had a "mail" system that is immediate. Never have we had too little time to prepare our own food. Never have we held phones to our ears 24/7. We are already beginning to learn of the consequences of some of these behaviors. What we are yet to truly realize en masse in the Western world is that the seeming urgency and the pace at which we are living is a disaster for human health, in particular our nervous systems. Not to mention the quality of the "immediate" food that goes along with this lifestyle.

We are so far removed from our origins that you can now eat a tomato in the middle of winter if you choose. As silly and insignificant as that sounds—and, of course, there are much more destructive food habits than eating a tomato in winter, as tasteless as they may be—it is a clear indication that we have lost touch with the guiding light of nature when it comes to not just our food but also our whole way of living. And in my opinion, Mother Nature knows best. Once, not so long ago, we treated colds with garlic and lemons. Now, we take a pill and hurry on. I could be on my soapbox for weeks! Essentially, it takes awareness and a commitment to eat with the seasons, even if you do so only some of the time, and it is certainly a challenge truly to rest in this age of immediacy. Yet rest we must.

We now ask our glands and organs, our livers, our gallbladders, our kidneys, our adrenals, our thyroids, our ovaries, our testes, our brains, and our digestive systems to cope with whatever we consume in our rush. There are, of course, consequences to this superfast pace of living and this book has been partly born out of my observations and reflections, as well as the science I have learned about what this period in our evolution is requiring of us.

We are not wired to cope with constant pressure, perceived or real, nor are we equipped long-term to eat poor-quality food and lead sedentary lifestyles, strapped to our computers, cell phones plugged into our ear sockets. As I said, this is the tip of a partially inglorious but incredibly fascinating iceberg and the Western world needs to ask, "Where to from here?" Let me remind you of what you already know.

. . . .

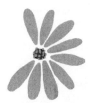

Introduction:
The Big Picture First

Accidentally Overweight is about what has to happen for a human to be able to access body fat and burn it. Essentially it is about weight loss and all the things that need to come together in our bodies to make it possible. The ultimate intention behind this book, however, is to free people from their battle with their bodies—a battle that may interfere with them sharing their full gifts with the world. Sound altruistic? Let me explain.

Whether consciously or subconsciously, many people are frustrated by how they feel about their body, or its appearance, and this frustration can take up headspace and influence their moods. This in turn can affect their self-esteem and the way they relate to the people around them. There are days when they feel fine, even quite good and positive, but the next day, or even later the same day, they feel revolting again, often for no obvious reason. They might feel heavy or swollen or sluggish or puffy or bloated or just plain yuck. When we feel this way, do you think we are likely to treat people—including ourselves and the people we love the most in the world—kindly or impatiently? Typically, it is the latter, and because those on the receiving end of your frustrations don't usually deserve the behavior you are dishing out, or understand the reasons behind it, they can easily interpret it with meanings that reflect how you feel about them, such as "he doesn't like me" or "she doesn't love me." Such unintended messages, and being on the receiving end of your impatience or sadness, can then go on to influence how they interact with others and feel about themselves. You can see how this vicious cycle can be perpetuated.

Furthermore, when we feel this way about ourselves, do you think we are likely to make excellent or poor food choices? Once again, the latter is the likely scenario, which of course only serves to compound our lousy view of ourselves. Yet, such a perspective is usually far from being at the front of our minds when we make such choices and so we just feel sadder and sadder about ourselves, including our appearance. We may feel like we will never be any different.

The other way I see challenges and frustrations with the body enormously affect a person's world is by the deep sadness that can develop—especially if they have, from time to time, made massive efforts to eat well and exercise regularly with little or no reward. Feeling like they are making no progress can drive their gaze inward and take up so much time and focus, again consciously or subconsciously, that they are unable to see that their body is, among many things, a tool through which they can learn. And the lessons on offer are those that can assist the individual as well the world around them. I've come to see that it is almost never about the body, just as it is never about the food. These are just the vehicles doing their best to wake you up. It is about a bigger picture. And once you've caught even a glimpse of that, let alone truly understood and integrated these insights, your relationship with your body, with food, with your health, and with the people around you will never be the same again.

Imagine waking up and your first thoughts *not* being about what you will or won't eat that day, or how much exercise you will or won't manage to do. Imagine not setting out to eat only this and this and this today but by 4 p.m. or thereabouts inhaling whatever you can get your hands on… and then berating yourself about how useless you are and that you have no willpower. Imagine not doing that ever again!

By exploring the physical mechanisms of your biochemistry and the emotional driving forces in your life, you will understand what has governed the growing and shrinking of your body up until now. And through that understanding and the practical solutions on offer to you throughout these pages, you will have your very own recipe to solve so much more than just your weight-loss puzzle. Food will no longer rule you, and your weight will simply fall into place. You will no longer measure or judge yourself by that magic number on the scales. In fact, there is every chance that you will stop weighing yourself altogether because you will naturally feel and look your very best, and you will know in your heart that you don't need a scale to validate anything about your beautiful self.

● ● ● ● ● ● ● ● ● ● ● ● ●

Digestion:
The Basis of Health

It never ceases to amaze me how magnificent and clever our bodies really are, and it astounds me how many processes go on inside the body without us having to give them any thought. Digestion is one of those processes. The nourishment we are provided, as a result of good digestion, is an extraordinary gift without which we would not survive. It is the process through which we get all of the goodness out of our food. Digestion is intricate and complex and yet relatively robust. And it is intimately connected to how you feel and function every single day, from the energy you feel to the fat you burn, from the texture and appearance of your skin to whether you have a bloated tummy or not, right down to your mood. Digestion is responsible for so much that goes on inside us. If this body system gives you grief, for example if you are bloated most evenings have intermittent diarrhea and constipation, or get reflux, you can reach a point where you feel like this is how life is always going to be. It must "just be how you are." Perhaps you believe it's "in your family." Well, bowel challenges do not have to be your reality.

Digestion is the essential place to start when solving your weight-loss puzzle. It is important that these initial building blocks to outstanding health are in place. It can be a challenge to balance hormones, for example, if your digestion is the bane of your life. The gut is essentially like a second brain in your body. Did you know that 80 percent of the body's serotonin is in the gut? And with serotonin being our primary happy, calm, content hormone, gut dysfunction can enormously affect our mood.

Some of the information in this section may make you giggle... it can be a bit tricky to find the right words to describe our stools! And some of the advice may at first seem obvious and too simple to make much of a difference. But reflect on your own eating habits and digestive system functions as you read on, and be ready to be accidentally overweight no more.

The digestive system

Digestion is the process of breaking down food so that we can absorb and utilize it for energy and nourishment to sustain our lives. Food is simply broken down into smaller components. For example, proteins are broken down into amino acids, and it is through this breakdown of food and the absorption of these smaller substances that we are nourished. As I have inferred, it is a process that never ceases to amaze me.

The digestive system is made up of a digestive tract, a big long tube (imagine it looking like a hose) and numerous ancillary organs, including the liver, gallbladder, and pancreas (figure 2 opposite gives you an idea of how it all fits together). The big long tube begins at your mouth, and food moves down the esophagus, through a valve, and into your stomach. The food then moves through a valve at the bottom side of the stomach into the small intestine, through the small intestine and ileocecal valve into the large intestine, and then any waste is excreted out the other end. When this process works well, you look and feel fantastic. When it is in any way impaired, the opposite can be true, and correcting it can change your life.

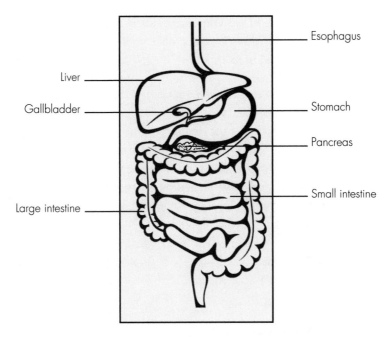

Figure 2: The human digestive system
The esophagus enters the stomach. From there, the
tube continues into the small intestine and then into
the large intestine; waste is then excreted. The liver,
gallbladder, and pancreas are also noted above.

Chew your food

Food enters the mouth and moves down the esophagus into the stomach. But what do we do to our food before it reaches the stomach? We chew it or, in some cases, we inhale it! There are no more teeth beyond the mouth. You can't chew it once the food has left your mouth. Yet, so many people eat as though their esophagus is lined with teeth. Many of us are in such a hurry with our meals, or we are so excited by the flavor of our food, that we might chew each mouthful four times if we're lucky. It's a case of chew, chew, chew, chew, mmmmm, yum, next forkful in, chew, chew, "Oh gosh my mouth is so full, better swallow some food..." So we swallow some partially chewed food and some not-at-all chewed food, and we do this day in, day out, year after year. And somehow we expect our stomach just to cope.

The stomach gets to a point where it doesn't like the rules by which you are playing anymore, so it takes its bat and goes home. Slow down! Chew your food! If you are a food inhaler, try this: Put food into your mouth, chew it really well, and then swallow it before you put in the next mouthful. I know that sounds simple, but try it. For food inhalers, it can take an enormous amount of concentration to change their eating behaviors. Put your fork and knife or spoon down between each mouthful if that helps. Engage in conversation if you are eating with others. Or, think of your own technique to slow yourself down if you hoover your food. You need to pay attention when you eat and to how you eat.

Watch portion size

Now back to the stomach, the first place your food lands after swallowing. Make a fist and look at it. Yes, clench your fist and observe its size. That is how big your stomach is without any food in it. Tiny, isn't it? So, think about what happens when you pile your plate high in the evening and inhale that big mountain of food. Your stomach has to stretch to accommodate it. And food has to sit in the stomach for a minimum of 30 minutes to allow the stomach acid and other digestive juices to begin to break the food down properly.

Once your stomach gets used to being stretched, it expects it every day, and this stretching is part of the reason why, if you decide to eat less or go on a "diet," you tend to feel hungry after your meals for around four days, as it can take a few days for the nerve endings around your stomach pouch to "shrink back" and become accustomed to smaller servings. The nerves are fired off when they reach a certain stretching point and send a message to the brain to let you know you have eaten.

This is one of the numerous mechanisms we have that has the potential to tell us to stop eating, that we've had enough. Trouble is, for some, the stomach is so used to being stretched, by the time the nerves fire, we may have overeaten and be berating ourselves. This is a process through which carbohydrates let us know we have eaten. With fat and protein however, once we have chewed these foods, messages are already being sent from the mouth to the satiety center of the brain to let us know we are eating. These signals usually reach the brain within five minutes of chewing, while the stomach stretch method can take more like 20 minutes! As an aside, it is important to include fats and/or protein with each meal, as you are likely to eat less and be satisfied with less total food for that meal than if you simply ate carbohydrate-rich foods on their own.

A rough guide to the amount of food we need to eat at each meal is approximately two fist sizes. That is concentrated (low in water content) food such as proteins or carbohydrates. You can and need to add as many greens (non-starch vegetables and/or salad) to that as you like. Although they have a high-nutrient content, they are mostly water. Remember that.

For some folks (not everyone), the key to body-fat management is simply eating less total food by reducing portion sizes. If this is you, make the decision to eat less. Reduce your portion size by one quarter, especially in the evening if you overeat, and see how you feel. Obviously, many people know they need to reduce their portion size or not eat after dinner, yet no matter how hard they try, they can't seem to eat less or stop eating once they start. This is why the "whys" behind our food/eating behaviors need to be explored and Puzzle Piece 9, Emotions, does just that.

Stomach acid pH

Food arrives at the stomach after you have chewed and swallowed it. The aroma of food, as well as the chewing action itself, stimulates stomach acid production, which is an exceptionally important substance when it comes to great digestion. The role of the stomach acid is to break down food. Imagine your food is a big long string of circles as shown in the first row of figure 3 below. It is the job of the stomach acid to go chop, chop, chop, and break the circles apart into smaller bunches, as the second row illustrates.

OOOOOOOOOOOOOOOOOOOOOOOO
↓ (stomach acid) ↓
OOO OO OOO OOO OO OOOO OO

Figure 3: Digestion
The action of stomach acid on whole foods breaks them down into smaller components.

Our bodies are governed by pH ranges, which is a measure of acidity or alkalinity. In scientific terms, pH refers to the concentration of hydrogen ions present, but you don't need to worry about that to understand this very important process. The pH range is based on a scale from zero to 14, with zero being the acid end of the spectrum and 14 being the alkaline end, while seven is neutral. Every fluid, every tissue, every cell of your body has a pH at which it performs optimally. The optimal pH of stomach acid is around 1.9, which is so acidic it would burn you if it touched your skin. But it doesn't burn you while it is nicely housed inside your stomach, as the cells that line the stomach itself not only produce stomach acid but are also designed to withstand the super-acidic conditions.

For many of us, though, the pH of our stomach acid is not acidic enough, and it may have a pH far greater than 1.9, which is not ideal for digestion. To be precise, animal proteins appear to be optimally digested at a pH of 1.9 while starch is optimally digested at a pH of 2.1; this may not seem like much number-wise, but inside your body, it can mean the difference between having a flat or a bloated abdomen after a meal. A professor in the USA has been researching the pH of stomach acid in various groups of people who have been diagnosed with specific conditions, such as children with autism spectrum disorder (ASD). Many children with ASD have been found to have a stomach acid pH of around four, far too high to be effectively digesting protein or starch.[1-3]

Adults with reflux or indigestion tend to assume that the burning sensation they experience with heartburn means they are producing too much acid, when the reality is usually the opposite. They are usually *not making enough* stomach acid and/or its pH is too high. To understand this, remember the analogy given above in figure 3, and that stomach acid plays a vital role in breaking the circles apart. A pH that is much higher than 1.9 cannot effectively break the circles apart and larger segments of, for example, seven circles in length may be the result. The body knows that if something that is seven circles in length continues along the digestive tract, it is not going to be able to further digest these partially broken-down circles. Rather than allowing that food to proceed down into the small intestine for the next part of its journey, the body regurgitates the food in an attempt to get rid of it. We then experience the acid burn and assume it is too acidic, when, in fact, it is not acidic enough to break down the food and allow it to pass into the small intestine. It "burns" you, because anything with an acid pH that is too acidic for the tissue to which it is exposed will create a burning sensation. When the acid is contained inside the stomach pouch, all is well, but when it escapes out of this area, the lining of the esophagus and the first part of the small intestine are not designed to cope with such acidic contents. Many people with reflux respond very well to the stimulation of stomach acid (and/or omitting problem foods for them) and experience much fewer symptoms as a result.

As described above, stomach acid is stimulated by chewing, and the aroma of food, as well as by the consumption of lemon juice and apple cider vinegar (ACV). The chewing action sends a message to the brain to send a message to the stomach to let it know that food is on its way. When we inhale our food, this doesn't happen. Historically, we regularly took much longer to prepare our meals and the slower cooking process generated an aroma of the upcoming meal, again signaling to the stomach that food was on its way. These days, many people aren't present when they eat. They watch TV or read a mobile device rather than looking at their food. Visual cues, as well as aromas, can help to support good digestion.

Lemon juice and ACV physically stimulate the production of stomach acid. If you haven't consumed either of these before, it is best to dilute them initially and ideally consume them five to 20 minutes before breakfast (or all of your main meals if that appeals). For example, you might begin with half a teaspoon of ACV in as much water as you like. Over the coming days and weeks, gradually work up to having one tablespoon of ACV while you gradually decrease the amount of water, or keep the larger dose more diluted. If you would prefer lemon juice, start with the juice of half a lemon diluted to your taste with warm water and gradually work up to having the juice of a whole lemon in less warm water. As an aside, it can be a good idea to wait for around 20 minutes to brush your teeth after you have consumed the lemon juice to prevent any potential problems with tooth enamel in the future. Use these tips to wake your stomach acid up before you eat!

The potential effect of drinking water with meals

We need the pH of our stomach acid to sit at around two. Water has a pH of seven (neutral pH) or above, depending on the mineral content (the higher the mineral content, the higher/more alkaline the pH of the water). When you add a liquid with a pH of seven or more to one with a pH of two, what do you potentially do to the stomach acid? You dilute it. And we need all the digestive fire we can muster to get the maximum nourishment out of our food and the best out of us. In my ideal world, we wouldn't drink water 30 minutes either side of eating.

When I'm giving a seminar on this topic, at this point in the presentation, a member of the audience invariably shouts out, "What about wine?" Wine has a more acidic pH than water, so although it puts a load on the liver (*more on pages 113–115 in Puzzle Piece 4, The Liver*), from a digestion perspective, it takes less of a toll than water. Usually, at that point in the seminar, I am everybody's new best friend!

You do not need to be concerned about the water content of food, nor do you need to focus on omitting all beverages at every mealtime. Simply aim to drink water between meals, not with meals, and don't put food in your mouth and wash it down with a swig of water. It can be a challenging habit to break. Set yourself a goal of not drinking with meals for one week... and then preferably keep the new habit going. Or, add a squeeze of fresh lemon juice if you insist on water with your meal for your own reasons. Just cut it out for a week, (one little week out of your very long life) and see if you feel any different.

PH gradient of the digestive system

Once food has been somewhat broken down in the stomach, it moves through the pyloric sphincter, a one-way valve leading into the duodenum, which is the beginning of the small intestine. Physically, in your body, this valve is located in the middle (or just slightly on the left) of the chest, just below where a woman's bra sits and just below a man's pectoral muscles.

While food is in the stomach, messages are being sent to the pancreas to secrete sodium bicarbonate (as well as digestive enzymes), which has a highly alkaline pH. The bicarbonate is designed to protect the lining of the first part of the small intestine, as well as allow digestion to continue. What is known as a "pH gradient" is established all the way along the digestive tract, and each region of the big long tube (*see figure 2, page 3*) has an ideal pH. When the pH gradient is not established in the stomach (i.e., when the pH is higher than ideal), digestion problems are likely further along the tract. These may be symptoms of the small or large intestine, such as bloating, pain, or excessive wind. It can also mean that the absorption of nutrients may be compromised. Insufficient pancreatic bicarbonate production may also cause digestive symptoms such as a burning sensation underneath the stomach in the valve area described above. Pain in this area can also indicate that the gallbladder needs some support or investigation. It is best to consult with your health professional about this if you feel discomfort in this area.

The best way to let the pancreas know that it needs to jump to action and produce bicarbonate and digestive enzymes is to have good stomach acid production at optimal pH. The digestive system runs off a cascade of signals from one organ or area to the next, via the brain. Use the suggested strategies given above, especially chewing food well, to stimulate the pancreas to fulfill its role.

There are occasions when I suggest clients use supplements of pancreatic enzymes, which are appropriate if there is a genuine lack rather than simply poor stomach acid conditions, but I usually suggest the aforementioned strategies *before* trialing supplemental enzymes. However, when symptoms are severe, and once other causes have been ruled out, a gastroenterologist might need to measure pancreatic enzyme levels.

Absorption

As food moves through the small bowel, digestive enzymes are secreted from the pancreas and the brush border (lining) of the small intestine. The role of these enzymes is to continue what the stomach acid began, which is to continue to break down the food we have eaten into its smallest, most basic components. It is in the small intestine where you absorb all of the goodness (vitamins and minerals) out of your food. Think about that. All of the goodness, all of the nutrients that keep you alive, are drawn out of your food and into your blood so that your body can use those nutrients to do all of the life-sustaining jobs it does. Alcohol and vitamin B12 are virtually the only substances you absorb directly out of your stomach (rather than your small intestine) into your blood. Alcohol tends to be in your blood within five minutes of consuming it, which is why humans may get tipsy if they drink it on an empty stomach.

The small intestine is where the nutrients in your food move from the tube that is your digestive tract into the blood, which is obviously a different set of tubes. This is how we are nourished, and it is how you stay alive!

Just because you eat something, though, doesn't mean you get all of the goodness out of it. Just because a food contains, for example, 10mg of zinc, doesn't mean you will get (absorb) the whole 10mg when you eat it. The absorption of nutrients is dependent on a whole host of factors, some of which have been discussed above. If you inhale your food, drink water with your meals, or have poor stomach acid production, for example, you may absorb very little of the goodness in your food. Nutrients are essential for life, so simply, as a result of the *way* you are eating, let alone the foods you might be choosing, you may be robbing yourself of some of the goodness your food provides. Give yourself the best opportunity to absorb as much goodness out of your food as possible by applying the tips above. It may add energy to your years and years to your life.

Is that niggling pain in your side appendicitis?

Countless clients describe experiencing on-again, off-again pain that hits them quite low down on the right-hand side of their abdomen. If you place your little finger on your right hip bone and use your thumb to find your navel, this pain tends to be located about halfway between on that diagonal line. This is the ileocecal valve, where the small intestine meets the large intestine. Many people mistake ileocecal valve pain for appendicitis, as the appendix is located close to this area. Always see a medical professional to diagnose your pain.

For many, pain begins in this area after a tummy bug (infection) or after travelling, usually overseas or camping, and having diarrhea, or after a bout of food poisoning. Even though the obvious symptoms of the causative infection have long since gone, it is as though the nasty little critters that caused the original upset tummy have taken up residence in the valve. Or perhaps they have changed its function. To remedy this pain, there are numerous options to try. One is to release the reflex connected to this valve by rubbing the area with your fingertips 20 times in an anticlockwise circular motion with reasonable pressure, not so it hurts you but also not with fairy fingers. Another option is to use anti-parasitic herbs, such as Chinese Wormwood and Black Walnut for four to eight weeks every day, before each main meal. The other potential remedy is one of my favorite substances on Earth, Lugol's Iodine, also known as Lugol's Solution. The liquid of potassium iodide is not only a source of iodine, necessary for so many body functions, but acts as a potent anti-parasitic agent that clinically seems to help clear the last of the nasty critters from this important valve. It is possible to overdose on iodine so it is best to check your dosage with a health professional to make sure the dose is right for you.

Gut bacteria

Now that the food has progressed through to the large intestine, can you guess what lives in here? Bacteria. On average, an adult will have 6½–9lb (3–4kg) of bacteria living in their colon. So, just as an aside, every time you weigh yourself remember that number on the scales is also comprised of gut bacteria that are essential for life. See how crazy it is that we weigh ourselves. All you do when you weigh yourself is weigh your self-esteem, but more on that in later chapters.

Some of the bacteria in your large intestine are good guys and some are bad guys. You want more good guys than bad guys. The role of the gut bacteria is to ferment whatever you give them. To come back to the circle concept of food (see figure 3, page 6), gut bugs love it when you give them something that is one or even two circles in size. They know what to do with that. But if a previous digestive process has not been completed sufficiently, the gut bacteria in our colon may be presented with fragments of food that are five or even seven circles in size, and all they know to do with any food they are offered is to ferment it.

What word springs to mind when you think of fermentation? I love asking this question at my seminars, as the answers usually amuse me as well as the audience. People will often say "beer," "wine," "sauerkraut"! But usually I get the answer I'm after, which is "gas." Fermentation involves bacterial action on a food source and the subsequent production of gas. Some gases are essential to the health of the cells that line our gut, while others seem to irritate them and give us a bloated, uncomfortable stomach as the day progresses, whether we have eaten in a "healthy" way or not.

The trouble with a bloated stomach for many women (in particular) is that it messes with their brain. When they look down and see a swollen tummy, something inside immediately communicates to every cell of their body that they are fat, whether they consciously think this thought or not. Many of my clients go up a size around the waist as the day progresses, even though they feel they have eaten with their health in mind. This can add a layer of stress to a person's life that they just don't need or understand. It is especially stressful because they can't fathom why it is happening. Sometimes it is the foods you are choosing. Sometimes it is the bugs that are living in your colon. Sometimes it is because of poor digestion further up the process, such as insufficient stomach acid. In Traditional Chinese Medicine (TCM), this is considered a spleen and/or liver picture and a TCM practitioner is likely to use acupuncture and/or herbs to support the spleen and liver.

Stress

Poor digestion can also be due to stress or, more precisely, adrenalin. Adrenalin diverts the blood supply away from your digestive processes and concentrates the blood in your periphery (your arms and legs). The reason for this is that by not having blood focused on digestion, you are more likely to get away from the perceived danger; it keeps you focused on escaping the danger. If blood were still concentrated on the digestive system, there is a risk you would be distracted by food. Again, if you really were in danger, which is what adrenalin communicates to your body, your life might be over if you suddenly spotted a piece of fruit hanging in a nearby tree rather than remaining focused on getting out of danger. Stress, stress hormones, and the processes they drive in your body, including those related to body fat, weight loss, and digestion, are explored in great detail later in this book.

Bowel evacuation

In dealing with clients one-on-one, I have had to work out ways to extract information from people using "appropriate" language and also with words that accurately investigate what is going on for that person. Many years ago, one of the questions I originally found difficult to phrase was around how empty someone felt after they had used their bowels. I tried to dream up ways to word this question so that it wouldn't make clients feel uncomfortable (not that many of them are concerned!) but also so that I could gain more insight into how their bowel was functioning. As with most things, a client turned out to be my teacher. While asking him about his bowel habits, he said, "You know what? My greatest discomfort comes from incomplete evacuation." There they were. The words I needed. So, early on in my consultation work with people, I started asking about feelings of incomplete evacuation.

For some, it's not an issue at all. They have no idea what I'm talking about when I mention it. For others, they are so excited that someone has finally given them the words to describe such frustrating discomfort. They wouldn't answer yes, if I asked them if they were constipated, as they may use their bowels every day. It is just that when they do go to the toilet, they feel like there is more to come but it doesn't eventuate and evacuate.

This feeling can be the result of numerous scenarios. It may be insufficient digestive processes as outlined previously. It may be inadequate production of digestive enzymes due to poor signaling or a damaged or inflamed brush border. It may be a food allergy or intolerance. It may be poor fiber intake or dehydration. It can be stress hormones causing the muscles surrounding the bowel to contract and hold onto waste. It may be a magnesium deficiency not allowing the walls of the bowel to relax and allow the thorough passage of waste. The thyroid gland may not be working optimally. TCM teaches us it may be insufficient spleen and/or liver chi (energy). The list of scenarios is almost endless.

One option to improve this challenge is to have a health professional help you get to the bottom (no pun intended) of it and remedy the situation. You might increase the green vegetables and decrease the processed foods in your diet for a week and see if that makes a difference, especially given that green vegetables are good sources of magnesium, water, and fiber, among other things. You may be suspicious of a food or a group of foods that are causing this feeling but because you love this food you are reticent to remove it. I cannot encourage you enough to remove your suspicious food from your diet for a trial period of four weeks. Four little weeks out of your very long life, an expression I use regularly with clients to highlight the relatively short time period necessary to offer potentially enormous insight into their health challenges. You may get an answer to your challenge over the trial period and, if not, you can relax and thoroughly enjoy this food that you love rather than silently wondering if it is the basis of your incomplete evacuation. But I can hear you already asking, "What if it works... what does that mean... can I never eat that food again?" My answer is always that it is your choice.

I've witnessed people be so resistant to dietary change but, after trialing a different way of eating, they feel so different, so much better that they have no desire ever to go back to their old way. I also meet others who miss a food terribly. If it is the latter, I suggest to that person, that "now they know." It is no longer a mystery to them why they feel this way. Then they are in control. Unless the problem is due to a true allergy, I find that when people are strong, meaning when they are very robust from a digestion perspective, their gut will tolerate this food better than if they are stressed. I also support them to explore why they feel they can't live without this particular food, as the reasons may also be emotional. Either way, once you know, you are in control, and it is your choice. You know that if you have an important event coming up, you might like to avoid the culprit food for a time so you feel and look your best for the occasion. Again, unless the food is a true allergy for you, your tolerance of it may change and improve over time, especially with a focus on gut healing and stress management. Don't think that because it hurts you today it always will. Your body changes and renews itself constantly. Just know there is a reason for your symptom. It is simply a matter of finding your answer.

One of the reasons I'm so concerned with bowel evacuation is that if this process is inefficient, waste can remain inside the bowel for too long. While it is there, it is fermenting. This can give the liver additional and unnecessary toxins to process, as well as "suffocating" the cells that line the colon. The waste can also dry out and harden, sticking itself to the lining of the bowel wall, narrowing the tube through which the new waste can flow. If you have ever seen soil in the middle of a drought, cracked, dried out, and unable to absorb a brief shower of rain, that is the way hardened feces can behave in your colon.

If this scenario occurs, waste can only move through the middle of this newly formed, feces-lined tube, and the efficiency of waste elimination is decreased. The old, hard, compacted fecal matter remains. When the cells that line the bowel are coated with hard feces, they are unable to "breathe," and a process that was once described in medical textbooks as "autointoxication" ensues. To remedy this, chamomile is one of the best things you can take. Drink plenty of tea, use the medicinal herbal tincture, or take capsules with each meal. Once the waste has dried out, it is difficult to rehydrate it so it can move through and be excreted. Chamomile softens the waste and helps the bowel wall relax. Drinking aloe vera juice before you eat breakfast can also be particularly helpful for an irritated gut.

Another remedy is one that many people have very strong opinions about: Colon hydrotherapy, or colonics as they are known. This process involves a tube being inserted into a person's rectum through which warm or cool water gently flows. This allows the hardened fecal matter to soften, like heavy, consistent rain on dried-out soil, allowing the large bowel to empty fully, often getting rid of built-up waste that may have been there for a very long time. I have had clients tell me that the waste they excreted during their first colonic was black, inferring that it may have been there for many years, interfering with healthy bowel function. I had a lady once tell me she saw popcorn in the "viewing" pipe during her colonic and knew that the last time she had eaten popcorn was at the movies with her ex-boyfriend whom she hadn't been with for over six months!

Colonics polarize people. The idea either appeals to you or it doesn't. There is no middle ground with people's love or dislike of colon hydrotherapy. I will encourage you, though, not to lose sight of what trends have done to medicine. Up until the early 1900s, colonics were part of general medicine, and doctors understood the importance of good bowel evacuation. When you examine the history of medicine and observe the split between what we now know to be Western medicine and complementary medicine, it is clear why this happened; however, this book does not seek to explore this segregation in detail. I will simply say that colonics were once accepted as a "normal" treatment method for a host of health conditions, not just bowel issues. With a well-functioning bowel, an enormous load is not only taken off the digestive system but also the liver, the organ primarily responsible for preventing accumulation of problematic substances in the body.

Help prevent bowel cancer by ensuring efficient bowel evacuation using methods that suit you! Always seek advice from a health professional before undertaking colon hydrotherapy, if it appeals to you.

Opioids

An additional concept within digestive health that is not only fascinating but also has wide-ranging effects on how we feel and function, including gut-transit time (how quickly food moves through the digestive system), mood, concentration, and, potentially, food addictions, is a concept known as the "opioid excess theory."

The cells that line a healthy small intestine look like a row of neatly stacked bricks with finger-like projections (called "villi"), side by side as demonstrated in figure 4 below.

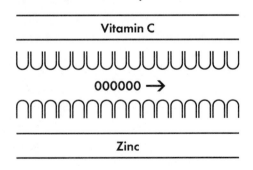

Figure 4: A healthy gut
Food (circles) traveling through a healthy mature intestine moves straight ahead. Only nutrients (e.g., vitamin C and zinc) enter the blood vessels that closely follow the intestines.

In a healthy gut, only the tiny nutrients (vitamins and minerals) diffuse (move) across the gut wall into the blood, and this is the precious process through which we are nourished and stay alive. However, the cells that line the gut can come apart, as if the bricks are stacked with gaps, illustrated in figure 5 below. This is, in fact, how we are born.

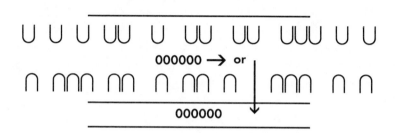

Figure 5: A "leaky" gut
Microscopic, poorly digested fragments of food (circles)
traveling through an immature gut or "leaky" intestine can
escape out of the gut and enter the bloodstream.

When we are born, the cells lining our digestive system are a distance apart, a primary reason why we can't feed all foods to newborns; foods must be gradually introduced to a child over time to prevent allergic reactions as the gut matures. The gut is immature when we are born, and it slowly matures from birth until reaching full maturity somewhere between the ages of two and five years, depending on the individual child and their health and life experiences in the early years. The cells lining the gut can, however, also come apart during adulthood as a result of a gastrointestinal infection or stress.

The chronic production of stress hormones can compromise the integrity of the gut cells and signal to them that they need to move further apart so that more nutrition can get through to the blood, as nutrient requirements increase during times of stress. Everything about us is geared for survival.

When food travels through a gut with good cell lining integrity, it can only go straight ahead. However, if it travels through a gut in which the cells have come apart, it may go straight ahead or move out of the gut and into the blood. Nutrients, the vitamins and minerals from food, are intended to enter the blood, not fragments of food itself. If the immune system, which protects you from infection, thinks that the food fragment is a germ, it will then mount an immune response against it. This is one way adults can develop food sensitivities. Poor gut integrity is also described as "leaky gut." Once you were able to eat anything without a problem, and now certain foods seem to cause you grief.

This process can be healed by minimizing the irritation to the gut lining by avoiding some foods or ingredients for a period of time, while also working on the gut integrity. Often people are able to tolerate the foods that cause them grief (if they choose to consume them) once we have worked out why they have the "leaky gut" symptoms in the first place. Did the problem begin as a result of stress or an infection? The power to heal the symptoms is always in the why. I seek to establish the road that led to the challenge for the patient, as the road in needs to be the road out.

The blood supply into which the food fragments flow is the same blood supply that goes to your brain. Humans have what is known as a blood-brain barrier (BBB), a semipermeable layer separating the peripheral blood supply from that of the brain. The BBB was always considered to be a highly selective membrane that only allowed substances into the brain that would be of benefit. Research has now shown us that this is not the case.[4] In cases where gut permeability is increased, the BBB is often suspected of having the same increased permeability. Further reading about this topic is noted in Resources and References at the back of the book.

If we could literally see the food fragments, their structure is very similar to that of opioids. Opioids are substances that help humans feel good and also modulate pain. We have our own natural feel-good hormones that have an opioid-based structure, called endorphins. In our brain and in our gut, we have what are called opioid receptors. Just because your body makes a substance (chemical messenger/hormone) doesn't mean you necessarily get the effects of that substance. The substance must bind to a receptor, just like a lock and a key fitting together, for you to get the effect generated by that hormone. In this case, when we make endorphins and they bind to the opioid receptors, we feel pleasure. Heroin and morphine are opioids and they too bind to the opioid receptors in the brain. Anything that gives a human pleasure has the potential to be addictive—hence, a human's capacity to be addicted to the aforementioned drugs. You can also see from this example how someone might become addicted to exercise. Activity certainly generates endorphins when we partake. So whatever brings you joy, whether it is a sunset, a spin class, a football game, or a child's laughter, what has happened in that moment is that you have made endorphins and they have bound to opioid receptors, and you have felt pleasure.

How does this relate to food? Some of the fragments of food that can escape out of a leaky gut into the bloodstream can also have an opioid structure. Their names include beta-casomorphine and gluteo-morphine. They are partially digested fragments of casein (a major protein in cow's milk products) and gluten (a major protein in wheat, rye, barley, oats, and triticale). Just like endorphins, these opioids from food also have the capacity to bind to the opioid receptors in the brain and very subtly make you feel good. The effect is not usually noticed as an enormous boost in mood, but you might feel like you can't live without this food, and have to eat it in some form daily or even at every meal.

I have found this to be the case countless times. If a patient has a set of symptoms that warrants omitting a food from their diet for a trial period to see if it will make a difference, some people have no problem; there is no resistance. Others will beg me not to exclude the food, even though they are seeing me because they want results, and all I am asking is for them to omit a particular food for four measly weeks, as that may just give them the answer to some of their health concerns! I am not judging someone who responds in this way. I am simply pointing out the power food can have over an individual can be just like an addiction. Their connection to it, their need for it, is often highly emotional and also potentially physical because of this opioid mechanism.

Food was never intended to fulfill this role for humans. Yet, on a physical level, it is possible that the opioid effect some foods have the potential to create (when a leaky gut is occurring), is one of the factors behind food addictions. This mechanism may be a reason why some people overeat or eat and feel like they can't stop. This is an area that deserves much more research, time, and money as the opioid excess theory may be involved in numerous health conditions as well as obesity. Much research has already been done in relation to children with autism and adults with schizophrenia where these "exorphins" (opioids from an exogenous source—consumed from outside as opposed to having been made by the body) have been found to play a role in the expression of symptoms of these conditions.[5] Food not only has the capacity to affect our body shape and size, but also our mood, and our digestion of some foods may be incomplete, leading to the generation of an opioid effect and addiction to particular foods. If you suspect this process is going on for you, omit all sources of that dietary component (gluten and/or casein) for a trial period of four weeks. The first four to seven days will likely be the most difficult, but persevere. The results may be enormously worth it. If you do omit significant dietary components from your diet for extended periods, it is important to consult a health professional to make sure you do not miss out on any nutrients essential for your health.

TCM perspective on digestion

The spleen rules digestion in TCM. TCM considers that each organ has its own vital energy, as well as there being whole-body energy.

If spleen energy is down, you will feel your usual hunger for meals, but as soon as you eat even a small amount, you will feel full and possibly bloated. Your short-term memory is likely not to be what it once was, and you may possibly feel as if you eat like a bird yet your weight continues to escalate. You can eat and exercise with a real commitment, but if your spleen energy is low, from a TCM perspective, your body fat may not budge.

Stimulating spleen energy can make a real difference. Acupuncture will do this, as will bitter herbs and warming foods. Bone broth can be particularly beneficial for healing the gut and is also nutritionally dense. You'll find more information about this and a recipe at www. drlibby.com.

Spleen energy will decrease in the first place from what is simply described as overthinking. The busy mind, relentlessly thinking of the next thing you need to do, takes energy away from the vital process of digestion every day, according to TCM principles. The spleen may also lose some of its strength if the liver or kidney (adrenals sit on top of the kidneys) energy is overbearing or low. Working with a wonderful TCM practitioner can also assist you to heal your gut.

Food combining

Food combining is not a dietary strategy I was taught at university. I share it with you here, though, as having worked with clients one-on-one now for more than two decades, I get to see what works and what doesn't work for people. And although science cannot explain the intricacies of why this approach helps some—not all—people significantly (I can hypothesize why it works), I include it here as a potential strategy to assist a digestive system that has a tendency to bloat and be unpredictable.

In clinical practice I've seen food combining enhance digestion, energy, vitality, and fat loss, and it can be a great way to combat a bloated tummy. It involves never eating animal protein with carbohydrate-rich foods. In practice, that means no meat with potatoes. No hamburgers in buns. It means that if you eat meat, chicken, or fish, you need to eat it with vegetables that have a high water content, not starchy ones, such as potato, sweet potato, pumpkin, corn, or any other starchy foods such as pasta, bread, or rice.

If you eat vegetable protein, such as one of the many types of lentils, chickpeas, beans, or tempeh then, under food-combining principles, you do not eat meat with these foods, but rather any vegetable at all, including starchy ones if they appeal. If you feel like eating rice then, with food combining, it needs to be a vegetarian meal. Seeds and nuts are also best eaten with vegetarian meals due to the vegetable protein content of the nuts and seeds. Based on food-combining concepts, oils and other foods rich in fats including avocado can be eaten with either animal-based meals or starch-based meals.

Another principle of food combining is that fruit can only be consumed as your first food of the day and not again during the day. You are also encouraged to omit all refined sugars, artificial flavors, colors, sweeteners, and preservatives. I know people who live by the concept of food combining and feel spectacular. I know others to whom it makes no difference.

If you want to try it, but it seems a little extreme, apply the zigzag principle. This means that most of the time you follow food-combining practices ("zig"), but one day a week—or two to three meals a week if you'd prefer—you relax and "zag." This way, food combining becomes a sustainable way to live, as you are able to socialize without feeling restricted and can also eat the foods you might love, just not every day. It is a structured way of eating on which some people literally thrive, and I have seen it truly change people's lives. For others, though, food combining would take every aspect of joy out of their lives. It is not for you if you feel like this. Use the zigzag principle if you do want to use food combining, or apply other strategies in this book to help support digestion or other pieces of your weight-loss—essentially your optimum health—puzzle.

Signs your digestive system needs support

- Reflux and/or indigestion

- Recurring bad breath

- Recurring bad taste in your mouth

- Recurring diarrhea

- Recurring constipation or faecal impaction

- Intermittent bouts of diarrhea and constipation

- Bloated, abdominal distension

- Excessive wind (based on your perception)

- Offensive odor to flatulence

- Pale stools

- Black stools

- Frothy stools

- Poorly formed stools (put simply, the ideal stool looks like a sausage)

- Food visible in stools

- Gut pain (all gut pain needs to be investigated by your doctor first)

- If you have traveled and had diarrhea (and this has ceased), but you haven't felt the same since

- Your tummy makes noises and you can hear them, particularly at night

- Unexplained fatigue (other causes ruled out)

- You feel lousy/worse after eating

- You regularly overeat

- You burp/belch a lot; even water sometimes makes you burp

- You feel like you are becoming sensitive to foods, or more and more foods

- You feel stressed regularly

- You experience what I refer to as "incomplete evacuation"

- You rarely feel hungry (and this is not due to overeating)

- You feel hungry. You start eating but then you feel full very quickly

- You feel "addicted" to some foods

- You take medication regularly

- You have taken antibiotics many times

- You tend to experience low moods

- You have been diagnosed with depression (80 percent of serotonin is made in the gut)

- You bowel habits are unpredictable

- Your skin is congested, breaks out easily and unpredictably, or tends toward redness/inflammation.

DIGESTION SOLUTIONS

Digestion is central and essential to every process in our bodies, which is why, although digestion is not a weight-loss puzzle piece on its own, I wanted you to read this section first, as it is the base from which we'll build. So, whether your focus is weight loss, optimizing your health and wellbeing, and/or improving a challenging or a diseased gut, understanding your digestive system is a crucial step on your way to exploring even more fascinating aspects of your health and solving your weight-loss puzzle.

• Slow down! Chew your food.

• Eat real food. Avoid processed food. Provide your body with what it has the equipment to digest.

• Include fats and/or proteins with each meal, as you are less likely to be hungry again quickly and more likely to easily eat less total food across the day, than if you simply eat carbohydrates on their own.

• If you worry that you don't eat enough vegetables for optimum health, focus on increasing your intake of plants. Whole foods are best. Or you can juice pure vegetables. Or make smoothies so you get the whole plant. You might prefer to use one small piece of fruit in these drinks initially for taste but aim to reduce the fruit content over time. Or if you travel or are busy, and making smoothies is not going to happen for you, use an organic green drink powder (usually made from ground-up vegetables) available from health food stores.

• Eat less. Reduce your portion size by one quarter, especially in the evening if you overeat, and see how you feel.

• Wake your stomach acid up before eating by using lemon juice in warm water or apple cider vinegar (ACV) before meals, breakfast in particular.

- Drink water between meals, not with meals.

- Use the strategies throughout *Accidentally Overweight* to ensure efficient bowel evacuation.

- Omit a food you feel you cannot live without for a trial period of four weeks. The first four to seven days will be the most difficult but persevere. The results may be enormously worth it.

- Use a herbal anti-parasitic if your digestion challenges began after a gut infection. This is best guided by an experienced health professional.

- Working with a wonderful TCM practitioner can also assist you heal your gut.

- Apply food-combining principles if this appeals and utilize the zigzag principle if that makes it more sustainable.

- Try aloe vera juice to start your day if you have a particularly irritated gut.

- Bone broth contains substances that can assist with healing gut integrity and is a nutrient-dense food.

- Look at your food while you eat it. Do not read or watch TV while you eat.

- Eat in a calm state.

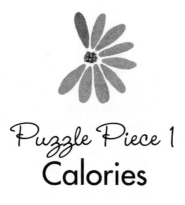

Puzzle Piece 1
Calories

Most of us have been taught that body shape and size are simply a matter of calories in versus calories burned. For many of us, in the early part of our lives at least, this appears to be true. Yet for some, eating less or exercising more may not seem to make the difference it once did, or perhaps ever did. For some, it makes no difference at all and no matter whether they put in maximum effort or zilch with food or exercise, their bodies remain overweight or in a state of constant expansion. People can be very quick to blame age, but if age were truly a factor then surely every 80-year-old would be overweight. Instead, what I have witnessed every day of my working life is the impact numerous body systems have on our metabolism—either as a result of lifestyle choices, life experiences, or pressure, whether real or perceived. Most frequently, all of these factors play a role. Only without emotion would our body shape and size be completely reliant on the calorie equation.

You know you need to eat less…

You cannot eat like a piglet and expect everything to fall into place. That's just common sense. You would have to have had your head buried in the sand for the past 30 years not to know we need to eat more fresh fruits and vegetables and fewer processed foods, and we all know it's not healthy to sit down all day. Yet I have met thousands of people who exercise frequently, often intensely—many even every day of the week—and still their body-fat levels don't change or, heaven forbid, they slowly increase. It saddens me to hear stories of people who have made a great commitment to eat well and exercise regularly, yet their bodies don't change. If you set out on your healthy regime to drop a clothes size and this doesn't happen, it can be disheartening. When that happens, people often throw all of their good intentions and better choices out the window. We forget about the other important benefits of exercise, such as improved bone density, lymphatic stimulation, clarity of thought, improved circulation, and, potentially, a deeper connection with nature, to name but a few. Just because we haven't dropped a clothes size or been noticeably rewarded for our efforts, we can easily wonder what the point is and give up.

Most humans are very black and white when it comes to food and exercise. Either we commit to regular exercise and eating well—choosing healthy meals and not much, if any, processed food or takeout—or we are sitting on the couch, not caring about what we put into our mouths, thinking to ourselves as we reach for the fourth chocolate cookie, "Oh, who cares, I've already blown it." For most people, real life happens somewhere in the gray area in between these two extremes. The problem is that even though we set out with a commitment to eat well and exercise regularly, too often we don't put an end date or review date on our plan.

Plenty of people make big decisions to eat well and exercise regularly only to find themselves, three weeks later, after a late day at work, buying takeout, polishing off a bottle of wine, falling asleep on the couch, and topping it all off by skipping exercise the morning after. Having made a decision three weeks ago to eat well and exercise regularly, most people will then berate themselves, feel like they have failed, and feel flat as a pancake in their mood. Yet if your best friend came into work the next day and described the challenging afternoon she'd had at work the day before, combined with the fact that she worked late, bought a takeout, polished off a bottle of wine, fell asleep on the couch, and didn't get up for morning exercise despite the fact that she'd told herself weeks earlier that she was going to eat well and exercise regularly… what would you say to her? Perhaps something along the lines, "Oh don't worry, you'll be all right. Today is a new day." Or perhaps something more like, "It was just one night, does it really matter?" Or "Did you enjoy yourself?"

Yet when *we* do it, we feel like it's the end of the world. And when you're buried up to your neck in guilt, feeling like it is the end of the world, are you more or less likely to make better food choices the following evening? Exactly. You're far more likely to do it all over again because you feel like you've ruined it. But you haven't ruined anything. If, on the other hand, you see what unfolded the night before as a part of life, or as already in the past, or good for your soul, you are far more likely to grin and then take better care of yourself the next night and get back into your movement the following morning. If you dig yourself into a hole filled with guilt, self-loathing, and frustration, it may be days, weeks, months, or even years before you step up and commit to looking after your physical health again. See the night before for what it was… one night—a "gray" night. This is part of real life for most people. And I can tell you right now that the guilt you feel and the harsh self-talk are far worse for you than any chocolate cookie will ever be. It is what you do every day that has an impact on your health, not what you do sometimes. You would never berate a friend the way you berate yourself.

Commit this statement to memory: *Without your health, you have nothing.* For so many, it takes a crisis before they sit back and reflect on what they've known for a long time: Lifestyle changes needed to be made. You're probably even thinking of whatever it is you need to change as you read this. Whether this change is to eat less sugar or drink less caffeine or alcohol, you know better than anyone. You don't need me to tell you. You know in your own heart when you are having too much of something and it is taking away from your health or quality of life. Make these changes now. Not tomorrow, not on Monday, right now. You know better than any health professional the changes you need to make. And as you continue through this book, different issues will begin to come up for you. As you read, things will fly into your head that are relevant to you. For example, you may know you need to eat less sugar, or perhaps you know that coffee doesn't suit you since it makes your heart race and you get the shakes when you drink it. If this is the kind of physical reaction you have, do you really think your body is saying to you, "Gosh, I'm glad you drank that"?

Your body does not have a voice. It can only give you symptoms to let you know whether it is happy or not. So pay attention to the signals your body gives you. Take reflux as an example. If there is a food that gives you reflux, think about what reflux is: You swallow some food and your body is bringing it back up. Do you really think your body is saying, "I'm so glad you just ate that, please eat some more"? No, it's expressing just the opposite! Your brain will sometimes try to override your body with comments such as, "Oh, but I love it, I can't *not* eat that food," convincing you that your love of a certain food is more important than any discomfort the consumption of that food may cause.

When it comes to food, we think in black and white. Your body isn't saying you're never going to eat this food again. It's simply saying, "Not right now, not today, perhaps not even next week— but *not necessarily* never again." Although, depending on the food, sometimes "never again" would be the best choice for your health and longevity! Reduce, or take a break from, the foods and drinks you know do not serve you well. Or only eat them when you know you are calm and able to eat slowly or when you are in great company. Keep in mind that it is what you do *every* day that impacts your health, not what you do sometimes, and see if that makes a difference. Support digestive processes in the ways suggested on pages 27–28 in the previous chapter and see if that makes a difference. But do not relentlessly continue consuming the food or drinks that drive your body to speak to you with negative consequences. No matter what, make an attempt to truly hear your body.

Food was designed to energize and nourish us. Yet many of us seem to have forgotten that. If you feel like you need to fall asleep after a meal, then that meal may not have served you (unless it was high in substances such as tryptophan, that actually induce sleep). Pay attention to how food makes you feel. Notice if a meal that is denser with protein or fats, or a meal that is higher in carbohydrates, energizes you or makes you feel lethargic. There is no easier time to do this than at breakfast. Does an egg at breakfast energize and sustain you? Or does it nauseate you? Notice these things. Does a grain-based breakfast, porridge, for example, sustain you through to lunchtime, or are you gasping for morning tea only an hour after you eat? Does porridge make you sleepy, or does it make you feel like you could run a marathon? Pay attention. Food is designed to energize you, not exhaust you. A great question to ask yourself before you eat is, "Will this nourish me?" This is something that can be answered from a nutritional perspective, which reflects on the food's vitamin and mineral content, or from a "soul" perspective. Sometimes eating (organic!) chips with a glass of (organic, preservative-free!) wine in the company of your dearest friends is the best thing ever. But, from my perspective, just not every day! You get the idea.

Sometimes you can't stop—emotional overeating

Finish this sentence: Food is...

For so many people, the type of word they use to finish this sentence is one relating to pleasure. For example, food is... delicious. Food is... amazing. Food is... yummy. If I ask an athlete that question, they will almost always say food is fuel or food is energy. My own response to that question is "food is nourishment." It is nourishment for my body, mind, and soul. A chef I know says food is love. A child I know says food is to make me big and strong. What's the point of this question?

If the answer is a word linked to pleasure, you are far more likely to over consume. My next question, if you answered with a pleasure word, would be to explore what else in your life currently gives you pleasure. Because if I am going to suggest you change the way you eat and, without realizing it, I suggest you avoid eating all the foods you link to pleasure, we need to help you identify activities or states of being that can replace the pleasure you find in that food, or you won't be able to stick to the plans we make. This is one of the main reasons diets don't work. Food is never the problem. It is the reason *behind* your poor food choices or desire for large portions that needs exploring and adjusting. Many of the people who have battled their weight for a long time don't believe they have easy access to other pleasurable thoughts or activities. Food is the easy option. Trouble is, pleasure on the lips is short-lived because deep inside they know what they are eating, or the way they are eating, is hurting them. They just don't know how to change it.

An athlete for whom food is simply fuel will rarely overeat to the point that it damages their health or performance. Granted, they may miss out on the pleasure that an appreciation of the combination of amazing colors, flavors, and textures on a plate can offer, but someone who views food as fuel rarely eats too much. For me, with the question "Will this nourish me?" the one I unconsciously ask before consuming anything (not that I realized this until I started working with people to help solve their health challenges), I almost always choose, without thinking, the nutrient-rich, real-food option, and I love every mouthful. In other words, the pleasure factor for me when I choose whole foods is enormous. I just don't consciously think about it. My subconscious focus is the nourishment. There are times, of course, when I will sit with some organic corn chips in a bowl while I look out across the ocean and, in that moment, the whole scene acts as nourishment for my soul. There is no guilt, no second thought about whether I made a good choice to eat corn chips—and my body size is not affected by a bowl of corn chips on the occasions I choose to eat them. I don't think like that. I pay attention while I eat. I notice and appreciate the crunch of every mouthful I take, and I'm focused on how grateful I feel for the vista in front of me.

This concept of being grateful and experiencing pleasure is important. If all I did was tell you to eat less, then, if you are a "food is pleasure" person, you may feel challenged to sustain this long-term. When you first change your diet and start eating nutrient-rich foods instead of processed, high-sugar, trans-fat laden non-foods, you need to be able to connect with, or focus on, something you are grateful for. It might be the shine in your child's eyes, your dog's playful nature, ears that can hear, eyes that can see, fingers that can touch, a nose that can smell, a roof over your head, or the magnificence of the day you are a part of... but focus on the things that light up your heart while you eat, and your brain will start to link your new way of eating to pleasure.

Some people know they eat too much. They know there is too much total food going in for them to be able to manage their body size, but—no matter how many promises of dietary change they make to themselves—they never seem able to follow through. They feel unable to control what they think is their appetite. Without them realizing it, this appetite for food is nearly always an appetite to feel differently, to feel an emotion other than the one wanting to rear its head. Yet at the time all they know is that they feel like eating lots of ice cream!

Say someone is eating too much—perhaps in the form of too many crackers with cheese before dinner, a big dinner itself, or a bucket of chocolate ice cream after dinner. If I meet with them for a one-on-one consultation and suggest they do this less often or not at all, they would do it for a period of time, partly because they had made an appointment to come and see me and they may have had to wait, they have paid me money for the consultation and so on, so there is a degree of commitment to the dietary changes we design. Because I've seen this pattern countless times, I use the consultation to begin immediately to discover whether the drive for the additional food is physical or emotional or, most likely, both.

On a physical level, chunks of cheese on way too many crackers may relieve dire hunger, yet if that person had eaten afternoon tea they would almost certainly be able to wait until dinner without inhaling a pre-dinner dinner of cheese and crackers. But with an inadequate lunch, or no afternoon tea, by the time they arrive home, many people's blood sugar is likely to be through the floor, something that makes most people feel like they could eat their arm off. Instead of that, they simply polish off way too many crackers and cheese. If your need is physical and fueled by low blood sugar then it is a physical pattern that we need to address.

But what could be an example of the emotional drive to eat? Eating when you can't possibly be hungry. Most of us know, of course, that eating a whole tub of ice cream after dinner is not only not good for our health but usually doesn't make us feel good by the time we have finished. Although you've eaten dinner, and on a physical level can't be hungry, you might still feel like you are. Perhaps you're in the habit of eating after dinner every evening, and every evening you go to bed feeling uncomfortable and lousy and berating yourself. Lying there in discomfort, you pledge that you won't overeat again tomorrow night. And in the morning you stand by your pledge. You eat very well all day. You don't snack before dinner—even though you feel like it—you eat your dinner, and then, not long after, you start thinking about ice cream. The argument begins in your head… "I'll just have one spoonful. Only one. Not the whole container. I know I said I wouldn't. But I really feel like it. What's one bite?" Something inside you knows that if you start, you won't stop. But still you start. You eat one, then two, and, before you know it, you are no longer thinking. And then the ice cream is gone. You've done it again. And then the self-loathing kicks in. You are bloated and uncomfortable, and you hate yourself. The situation seems hopeless. After nights, weeks, years, or even decades of discomfort, you feel as though you will never be able to stop eating, and you feel as if you will never be able to lose any of your body fat. You tell yourself you have no discipline, yet you need to remember that all you are doing is meeting an emotional need.

Trouble is, many people are unaware of how they really feel or would prefer to deny the anger or sadness, for example, which is just below the surface. Their perception is that it is "safer" not to acknowledge it. We are governed by how we feel and our every drive is for survival.

Understanding why you overeat

We will explore emotions later in the book. In this chapter, I simply wanted to show you a number of different scenarios through which excess calorie intake, no matter what the cause, can be the piece of your weight-loss puzzle that needs the most attention. I also want you to open up to the idea that emotions may be at the heart of why you overeat, so the emotions piece of your puzzle may also be highlighted.

Taking in too many calories is not the only reason some people cannot lose weight. Indeed, some people eat beautifully from a calorie perspective and exercise regularly, yet their body doesn't seem to change. On a physical level, this may be due to a variety of body systems, such as the production of stress hormones, the balance of sex hormones, liver function, gut bacteria profiles, thyroid function, insulin, leptin hormone levels, exercise methods, and the nervous system. Any or all of these systems can play a role when people do all they can for little or no reward.

The messages in this book do not deny that willpower has a place. Of course it does. My concern is that for people attempting to lose weight, it has been their backstop of blame. They can see no other reason other than a lack of willpower for what they classify as their failure to achieve a smaller body. But it's important to remember that we are geared for survival, and the hormonal systems outlined above know that better than any ounce of so-called willpower you can muster. If your body believes that your life is in danger, it will act accordingly; and sometimes that means fat storage, despite your best efforts. This will all make sense as you see how the pieces of your puzzle fit together.

For some, eating less is as simple as making the decision. That's it. No more overeating. They make the decision and follow through with great eating behaviors, and excess body fat is never an issue for them again. They may simply change their minds and begin to take good care of themselves, with outstanding nutrition and regular, functional movement. For others, however, it doesn't feel as simple as making a decision. They know they "should" make a change, but it feels too hard or as if they've already "tried" everything. Some people feel that they make an effort every day and are never rewarded. So, are calories one of the pieces of your weight-loss puzzle that needs attention?

Signs the calorie piece of the puzzle needs addressing

- You know you need to eat less but can't seem to do it yourself

- You have tried every diet!

- You are either on a diet or off a diet; you find living in the gray difficult when it comes to food and exercise; it's all or nothing

- You count calories and in your heart you know that you obsess about this or your weight

- You sometimes start eating and feel like you can't stop

Please note, you will also likely need to explore thoroughly and apply the strategies in the Emotions chapter (*see page 179*).

CALORIE SOLUTIONS

If the calories piece of your weight-loss puzzle has been highlighted for you, whether you think it's due to purely physical or emotional needs, or a combination of both, consider implementing the tips below.

- Serve dinner on a smaller plate.

- Eat two fist sizes of food (concentrated food such as protein and/ or starch) as well as plenty of greens with a high water content for most of your main meals. Snacks can be up to the size of one fist.

- Do not weigh food.

- Do not ever weigh yourself; you simply weigh your self-esteem and set yourself up to feel stressed and/or miserable over the day if you start your day this way. You know by the way your clothes fit you if your size is decreasing. Start to focus on how you feel, and work on feeling better and healthier rather than weighing less. A feminine essence responds to praise while a masculine essence responds to challenge. For many women, scales don't praise them and so don't inspire them. For many men, if they don't weigh what they want to weigh, their response is "I'll just work harder."

- Get some discipline around your thoughts. You are more likely to make poor food choices when you are (silently) saying mean things to yourself.

- Eat slowly.

- Chew each mouthful a minimum of 20 times.

- Chew each mouthful and swallow before you put the next mouthful in.

- Eat regularly; don't get ravenous so you feel like you want to eat your arm off.

- When you are first making changes, set short-term targets for yourself. If you eat takeout most days, you could try starting with "I am not going to eat any takeout until Friday, and then I can have whatever I like." Or if you don't usually eat many vegetables, commit yourself to eating vegetables for six out of the next seven nights. Perhaps you drink too much sugar because of the wine or soda you consume? In that case, decide to drink these beverages only on Friday or Saturday, rather than every night. It is also important to reflect on how you feel when you follow through with what you say you will do. Commend yourself—but not with a food or drink reward. Look yourself in the eye and tell yourself you are proud of yourself. You may feel a trifle foolish at first, but persevere until you can hold your gaze as you say the kind words to yourself.

- Allow some short-term targets to stretch beyond a week to two weeks.

- Remind yourself that you keep your word in your commitments to other people, so it's time to show yourself that you truly care about yourself and keep your word for these short bursts of time. As you explore in this book the other factors that influence body fat, you will begin to see there is much you can do to change your desire for food in the first place.

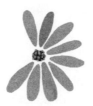

Puzzle Piece 2
Stress Hormones

Your adrenal glands are two very precious walnut-sized glands that sit just on top of your kidneys. They may be small in stature, but the power they pack when they are working optimally is an energetic gift to us all. The adrenal glands produce many hormones, two of which are your stress hormones, namely adrenalin and cortisol.

Adrenalin and the big sugar rush

Adrenalin is your short-term stress hormone. It is your acute stress hormone, the one that's produced when you get a fright. If someone suddenly runs into the room and startles you and you jump, that feeling that most of us know very well is caused by adrenalin. Adrenalin is designed to get you out of danger—and fast. Historically, we made adrenalin when our life was being threatened, and our response, fueled by adrenalin, was typically physical. A tiger might have suddenly jumped out of the jungle at us or perhaps a member of another tribe came running towards us with a spear. In that moment, you made adrenalin to get out of danger. Adrenalin promotes what is known as the "fight-or-flight" response. When activated, the typically excellent blood supply to your digestive system is diverted away to your periphery, to your arms and your legs. This is necessary because you need a powerful blood supply to these muscles to get you out of danger.

You also need fuel to give you the necessary energy, and the most readily available fuel is glucose—often referred to as sugar (a carbohydrate). Your liver and muscles store glucose in the form of glycogen, and adrenalin communicates to your liver and your muscles that energy is required. They then convert glycogen back into glucose and dump this glucose into your blood. Your blood sugar subsequently shoots up, ready to fuel your self-defense or your escape.

This cascade of events—and the biochemical changes that result— allows you to escape from danger in a very active way. Regardless of the outcome, regardless of whether you win that challenge or not (you escape, die, or win the fight), this stress, the threat to your life, and the need for adrenalin, is over very quickly. The trouble is that for many of us in the modern world, it is more often psychological stress that drives us to make adrenalin. And so although our life may not literally be threatened, this hormone still communicates to every cell of our body that our life is indeed at risk.

Psychological stress can come in many forms. It may be that you return from a two-week break at the beach to find 800 new emails in your inbox, and you wonder when on earth you're going to find the time to deal with those. It may be that your landline rings and, while you take that call, your mobile rings, and you feel that you can barely finish one conversation before having to start another. It could be that you set your alarm for the morning, you press snooze... you keep pressing snooze and suddenly you sit bolt upright in bed and realize you're running late. You may still have to iron clothes, prepare lunches, and deliver little people to school and, because you're leaving later than usual, you get stuck in traffic. Meanwhile, your mobile phone starts ringing with people at the office wondering where you are as you are supposed to be in a meeting, but you are stuck in the middle of rush-hour traffic, and your brain has gone into overdrive with the enormity of your morning. And you've only been up for an hour!

When you finally burst through the doors at work, all you can think about is how much you want a coffee. So all morning you've been making adrenalin, and now you are going to make even more adrenalin, as caffeine promotes its production. All you actually want from the "coffee" at this point in your day is a little breathing space. The reasons we crave a hot drink may vary, but often it's just to catch our breath. In those coffee-break moments, there is a bubble around us, and we are silently communicating, "Don't you dare come near me for the next three minutes!"

One important difference between the past and modern day is that the biochemical changes generated by adrenalin, such as sugar being dumped into your blood to get you out of danger, serve a useful purpose while you are physically fighting or fleeing. However, if you're sitting on your bottom at your desk in front of a computer and sugar is being dumped into your blood, you make insulin to deal with that elevation in blood sugar. And insulin is one of our primary fat storage hormones, as you will see in later chapters.

How coffee can make you fat

I know. Some of you will want to block your ears at this information. Sorry, it's just part of our biochemistry. Caffeine acts on the adrenal glands by stimulating the production of adrenalin. When adrenalin is released, your blood sugar elevates to provide more energy, and your blood pressure and pulse rate rise to provide more oxygen to the muscles, which tense in preparation for action. Your pupils also dilate to see more in less light, and your immune function stops firing as, from the body's perspective, fighting infection is not essential at this unsafe point in time. Blood is diverted away from digestion, and reproductive functions are down regulated since they use a lot of energy and are not necessary for our immediate survival, given the impending threat. Plus, your body does not believe it is "safe" to bring a baby into what your body perceives is an unsafe world. Not when your stress hormones are telling your body that your life is in danger (adrenalin) or that there is no more food left in the world (cortisol)!

Whether your adrenalin production is the result of real or perceived stress, or simply the result of your caffeine intake, caffeine, via stress hormones and coupled with the response of your nervous system (explored later in detail), can either lead you to slenderness or fat storage, because insulin—the fat-storage hormone—will firstly convert unused glucose from your blood into glycogen and store it in your muscles and what is left over will be converted into body fat. Let me explain this with the story of a client I'll call Anne.

Case Study

Anne, a strikingly slim and physically beautiful woman, had an appointment to see me. I did what I do with every client, and asked how I could help her and what she would like to get out of our session. Anne apologized for what she thought would sound vain and said that she had gained 7lb recently and was seeing me because nothing in her diet or activity level had changed to which the weight gain could be attributed. She was concerned that she might be perimenopausal even though her periods had not changed. She said some of her friends had gained weight during perimenopause, and she was here because she was concerned that it would become 20lb before she knew it, if she didn't get to the bottom of why her body had changed. I admired Anne's attitude and her desire to understand her body better. We discussed the many facets of her life, emotional and physical, and when it came time to talk about her food, her diet was truly amazing with regards to all of my benchmarks of eating a diet based on real foods.

People like me have numerous strategies (as you will see) that we can apply to assist someone in their quest for fat loss; from a food perspective this lady was already living by all the tricks of my trade. When it came time to talk about her liquid intake, she politely informed me that she had one glass of red wine four times per week and that she had done this with her husband for years. And then I asked if she drank coffee. Anne's eyes lit up. She replied that, yes, she loved it, but acknowledged, on reflection, that her caffeine intake was something that had changed. She had always had a coffee before breakfast every day for most of her adult life, and that was the only caffeine she consumed all day. But for the past three to four months, she had begun to have up to four coffees per day, but she didn't know why. She just had. When my eyes lit up back at her, she quickly justified her intake by saying, "But they are all black coffees, so there are no calories in them." She drank them all at her desk. She had never exercised, and I could see she had very little muscle mass. Her body fat, she said, had gone on around her tummy.

Anne could see from the look on my face where I was about to go and, before I'd even spoken, said "Please don't take them from me." I wanted her to see how emotionally attached she was so I didn't interrupt her. Eventually, I said that I believed it was the coffee that had led her to gain her 7lb, and she cried. She told me it was impossible, and she kept coming back to the calorie reasoning. She virtually had a tantrum in my office. I gently tried to lead her to the truth that actually it's only a drink, yet she behaved as if her four daily coffees held the meaning of life for her. I then went on to explain the mechanism I outlined above involving caffeine, adrenalin, elevated blood sugar, and subsequent insulin production. I told her that I wasn't even asking her to give up caffeine entirely. My clients will tell you that, when it is warranted, I often ask them to give up caffeine completely for four weeks. They are often shocked by how much more energy they have without caffeine in their lives. I simply wanted this client to go back to her one cup a day before breakfast, a coffee prepared with love by her husband for her. Anne agreed to make this change for four weeks, even though she couldn't imagine anything being more powerful than calories in fat creation and couldn't see how this plan could possibly work. I did nothing else for this woman.

Not one other change to her dietary intake and, four weeks later, she burst through my door telling me she had lost 9lb in four weeks, more than she had gained in the first place. I have never weighed a client nor will I ever weigh a client. My theory was that Anne's weight gain was the result of the perception of her nervous system, rather than the result of too many calories. Her subsequent weight loss was, in my opinion, extremely fast, but my point in sharing this story with you is to demonstrate caffeine's power to signal what is, for some, fat storage. Granted, this will not happen for everyone. It is significantly dependent on, as I mentioned earlier, the balance of your nervous system (discussed in detail in later chapters).

• • • • • • • • • • • • • • • • • •

So consider your caffeine habits and get honest with yourself about how it affects you. Does it dull your appetite and so unconsciously you grab a coffee instead of eating? This is especially true for many women at lunchtime. Does it make your heart race, give you the shakes, or loosen your bowels? Does it elevate your blood pressure? Or does it nourish your soul with no ill effect whatsoever? You know yourself better than anyone. Act on what you know is true for you.

Think about all of these mechanisms. So many of us run on adrenalin. Moment to moment, day to day, it's like a light switch has gone on, and it hasn't entirely switched off for a really long time. And it doesn't have to be traumatic stress and shocking situations that drive this process in us. It can simply be the pace at which we live our lives; the juggling act that leads so many people I meet to say that they want more "balance" in their lives. Some people even seek the feeling adrenalin gives them, and they only feel like they are living when adrenalin is pumping through their veins.

The human body is incredibly resilient, and although we were not designed to withstand long-term stress (due to the way we're designed, we are healthier when it is short-lived), many bodies appear to tolerate, as opposed to thrive on, years and years of living on adrenalin. Part of the challenge, however, is that once your body perceives that the stress has become long-term, your stress hormone output patterns can begin to change, presenting new—and often undesirable—changes to the body.

Cortisol—friend or worst nightmare?

Cortisol is your long-term stress hormone. Historically, our only long-term stress revolved around food being scarce. Long-term stress came in the form of floods, famines, and wars. During such times, we didn't know where the next meal was coming from. Today, in the Western world, our long-term stresses are more likely to be financial stress, relationship concerns, and uncertainty, or even worries, about our health, or the health of a loved one, but also body weight. For so many people, their first waking thoughts involve, "What will I or won't I eat today?" or "How much exercise can I get done today?"

Or, for some, the thoughts might flow like this: "Oh, my goodness, it's Wednesday, and I still haven't been to the gym, and, my gosh, it's 7 p.m. and there's no food at home, which means I still have to go grocery shopping, and that means I won't get home until 8:30 p.m. and then I have to cook and clean up and then it will be midnight before I get to bed and I have to get up at a good time to get to work early in the morning, but I'm going to a party in three weeks and I really wanted to fit into my favorite red dress and that's not going to happen because I haven't been to the gym all week and I am still not going to go tonight because otherwise I won't get any sleep and get to work on time to do everything I have to do..." And on and on and on it goes. Phew! So many people live like this most days of their life, whether they reveal it in how they live or simply think it. When it happens day after day it can easily lead to a chronic pattern of stress response, hence increased cortisol output, which in turn can lead to a change in your metabolism.

It is important to understand how cortisol works, as it can be your friend or one of your worst nightmares! When made at optimum amounts, cortisol does numerous wonderful things for your health. It is one of the body's primary anti-inflammatory mediators, meaning that wherever there is inflammation in the body, cortisol, having been converted into cortisone, dampens down the effect of that inflammation and stops your body from feeling stiff, rigid, or in pain. Many people, for example, will describe feeling that they have suddenly aged when they come out of difficult times. In the right amount, cortisol is not only an anti-inflammatory, it also buffers the effect of insulin, meaning that optimum amounts help you continue to burn body fat for energy while also maintaining stable—as opposed to rapidly fluctuating—blood glucose levels.

Cortisol levels change over the day and the right amount assists various bodily functions. Cortisol is designed to be high in the morning and, for the purpose of this discussion, let's say that 25 units at around 6 a.m. are ideal. Cortisol is one of the mechanisms that wakes you up in the morning and helps you bounce out of bed full of energy and vitality. By midday, optimum cortisol will sit at around 15 units, and by 6 p.m. levels will ideally be at around four units. By 10 p.m. in the evening, optimum cortisol levels are around two units, a level at which they are designed to stay until around 2 a.m. when they slowly and very steadily begin to rise again.

Figure 6 below shows the changing amounts, and it is true what your mother told you: one hour of sleep before midnight is worth two after, because cortisol starts to rise around 2 a.m. and the waking up process gradually begins. Do you ever wake up around 2 a.m.? Continue reading, for it may be related to your adrenal glands, your liver… or both!

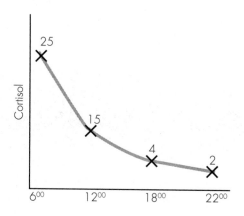

Figure 6: Optimal cortisol profile
Cortisol is nice and high in the morning and falls away again by the evening.

As a stress response continues, the effect on the body begins to change. In the early stages of stress, one of the first challenges cortisol presents is that the evening level of the hormone starts to spike again rather than continuing to decrease. At this stage, you still make optimum levels in the morning and are able to bounce out of bed and get on with your day with reasonable energy, but evening levels are creeping up. This is one mechanism through which good sleeping patterns can be challenged.

When cortisol levels become elevated above optimal, other changes in body chemistry begin to unfold. It has been suggested that elevated cortisol is the one common thread behind what we have come to describe as metabolic syndrome; that is elevated blood pressure, elevated cholesterol, and insulin resistance, the latter condition being a warning sign that if nothing changes in the near future, Type 2 diabetes is a likely consequence. If we remember that we are completely geared for survival and that cortisol tells every cell of the body that food is scarce, another of its roles is to slow down your metabolic rate. A slower metabolism leads you to burn body fat for energy far more slowly then you have in the past, as cortisol is designed to make sure that you survive this perceived period of famine.

Cortisol is "catabolic," meaning that it breaks proteins down into its building blocks, known as amino acids. Your muscles are made from proteins, and cortisol signals them to break down, as the body's perception is that fuel is needed. Additional amino acids are also needed in the blood to help repair tissues (even though you may be simply sitting in front of the TV, with your financial or relationship concerns mulling around your head!). The amino acids released as a result of the catabolic signaling of cortisol can be converted, through a process called "gluconeogenesis," back into glucose (sugar), which your body thinks may be useful to assist you in your stress. Yet if you're not active, this increase in blood glucose will not be utilized, and insulin will have to be secreted to return blood glucose levels to normal by returning the glucose in the blood to storage. Remember that glucose is stored as glycogen in the muscles and the liver.

But over time, the catabolic signaling of cortisol itself may have broken some of your muscles down, so now there is less space for glucose storage. As a result, some of the blood glucose returns to the remaining muscles while the leftovers are converted into body fat. Keeping the glucose level of the blood within the normal, safe range is of more importance to your body than whether you have wobbly bits around your middle! Essentially, too much cortisol can make you fat through dysregulated blood-sugar metabolism, not just fat metabolism itself. This is also a process through which long-term stress can lead to Type 2 diabetes.

Because cortisol is produced when stress has been going on for a while, your body (not knowing any better) thinks there is no more food left in your world, and it instinctively knows that it has a greater chance of survival if it holds on to some extra body fat to get you through the lean times. In modern times, when, for health reasons or vanity (or both), many people understand the importance of not carrying too much body fat, cortisol can provide a potential challenge to someone who believes that eating less is their only solution to body-fat loss.

Understanding the cortisol problem

If cortisol tells every cell of your body that food is scarce, and your metabolism slows down as a result, and you continue to eat and exercise in the same way you always have, your clothes will slowly get tighter. With cortisol telling every cell in your body to store fat, it is very difficult, if not impossible, to decrease body fat until the cortisol issue is resolved. We must get to the heart of the stress and either change the situation or change the perception.

Cortisol has a very distinct fat deposition pattern. You typically lay it on around your tummy, and, once again, the reason for fat placement here is governed by the body's quest for survival. If food suddenly ran out, your major organs need protection and warmth, plus they have very easy access to fat (fuel) that will keep you alive. You also tend to lay fat down on the back of the arms, and you grow what I lovingly call a "back veranda." To reiterate this important point: What do most people do when they notice that their clothes are getting tighter? They go on a diet, and, when you go on a diet, do you tend to eat more or less? You typically eat less (although some audience members call out "more" when I ask them this question at an event!), and in doing so you reaffirm to your body that food is scarce. But food is not scarce. It is abundant for you. If you want a chocolate bar at 3 a.m., you can get one. Eating less on your diet confirms to your body what it perceives to be true and that slows your metabolism even further.

Another challenge you face with elevated cortisol coursing through your body is that, since your body thinks that food is scarce, any time you see food, it's very easy to overeat, no matter how firmly you intend to eat only three crackers when you get home from work! If that packet of crackers is open and in front of you, cortisol will scream at every cell of your body, "You are so lucky! There's food there! Eat it!" and somehow, before you know it, the whole box of crackers is gone. Please don't get me wrong... I am not saying that self-discipline and willpower have no place. My intention is simply to point out that we have very ancient hormonal mechanisms in action inside our bodies that believe they know better than you when it comes to your survival. Your body can be your biggest teacher if you learn how to decipher the messages it is communicating to you. And extra body fat is sometimes simply a vehicle of communication.

Silent stress

What about when the stress is silent? You might not be a drama queen running around, arms flailing all over the place, screeching, "I'm so stressed, I'm so stressed!" You may be a very private person and keep things mostly to yourself. You may be so private with your fears and concerns, only presenting a happy face to the world, that you don't even realize that you're worried about things or that you may have been in a stressed state for a very long time.

When you feel grateful for the life you have, it's very easy to feel guilty if you complain about anything. A common internal phrase will be, "There are so many people worse off than me." This thought immediately makes you feel guilty and you stop focusing on your source of stress. Trouble is, although there *are* people worse off than you in this world, the minute you feel guilty, you change your focus so you don't ever get the opportunity to identify what is really bothering you and, more importantly, *why*. These "whys" are explored in detail later in Puzzle Piece 9, Emotions. For now, I'll share a common example, one that involves keeping the peace, to help you determine if cortisol, from an emotional source, is a likely piece we need to solve in your weight-loss puzzle.

Basic psychology teaches us that humans will do more to avoid pain than they will ever do to experience pleasure. Some people I meet will do anything, for example, to keep the peace and avoid conflict. Inwardly they become highly strung because they are always walking on eggshells around others, usually their intimate partner. "Hello, silent stress hormone production!" Others avoid feeling emotional pain by eating too much or making other poor food choices; perhaps by drinking bucketloads of wine or chain-smoking cigarettes. Alternatively, some people might write in a journal, go for a walk, a run, or a swim, while others will phone a friend and chat to deal with emotional pain. And all of these activities may take place with no conscious understanding of why.

Worrying can make you fat

You think you want to lose weight more than anything? You think you would do anything to be slimmer? You probably already have all of the information you need to do this. So what's stopping you? Or what stops you once you've started?

Every day of my working life, I meet people who eat too much. They know they do, but they can't seem to stop. Sometimes it is nutritious food, sometimes it's not, but, whatever the case, they know they would be much better off if they ate less or chose better-quality food.

Often these people are seeing me because they want to lose weight and they are precious, intelligent people who don't understand why they do what they do. These people know what to eat and what not to eat to lose weight, yet they don't do it, even though they truly believe that they are desperate to lose weight.

There is a really big difference between eating two squares of chocolate and eating the entire block, between one cookie with a cup of tea in the evening and eating a dozen. We all know that eating too much makes us feel full and uncomfortable, but, worse, it usually drives us to say very unkind things to ourselves such as, "I'm so useless, I have no willpower," and we go to bed feeling guilty and sad and believing we will never be able to change. The belief that things are permanent is very destructive.

So what might be going on for someone who, even with good intentions, just can't stop eating? Besides elevated cortisol due to long-term stress, there may be other biochemical factors involved such as low progesterone, poor thyroid function, or blood sugar that surges and plummets. There are also likely to be emotional factors (explored in Puzzle Piece 9, Emotions) and core beliefs they probably aren't even aware of, something I guide participants to explore thoroughly at my weekend events. Witnessing their "a-ha" moments is an honor.

One of the most wonderful and helpful statements my mother ever made was, "Don't worry about something until it's a problem." If it becomes a problem, then you can face it, but worrying about something that truly may never happen only serves to hurt you. As we now know, stress, whether it is real or perceived, may promote the production of excess cortisol. The ripple effect of a worry can very slowly and subtly change your metabolism to one of fat storage and a headspace of sadness and withdrawal. And it's the chemical signals of your body that are driving this. The beautiful piece of wisdom is useful to remember and act on, especially if you are a worrier:

'God, grant me the serenity to accept
the things I cannot change,

Courage to change the things I can,

And the wisdom to know the difference.'

THE SERENITY PRAYER BY REINHOLD NIEBUHR

Adrenal fatigue

The next biochemical stage of stress that can occur, especially if the stress has been prolonged, may involve cortisol falling low. If you have had a high level of cortisol output for many, many years, your adrenal glands may not be able to stand the tension, or have the resources to sustain such continual, high-level cortisol output and the metabolic consequences this drives. The adrenal glands were never designed to maintain this pattern of production and so cortisol output plummets. In general terms, you "burn out." In more recent times, this has become known as adrenal fatigue, because the major symptom is a deep and unrelenting fatigue.

Cortisol is supposed to be high in the morning, and ideal amounts help you bounce out of bed. It plays a role in how vital you feel and helps the body combat any inflammatory processes that want to kick in. Stiffness is a key symptom of adrenal fatigue.

For those with chronic stress, morning cortisol levels tend to be low, and, if 25 units is the ideal, with adrenal stress you may only get to 10 units or fewer. It can be very difficult to get out of bed with such low levels. By mid-afternoon, it will be at an all-time low, and you feel you need something sweet, something containing caffeine, or a nap to get you through your afternoon (this can also be the result of low blood sugar, which is covered in detail in Puzzle Piece 7, Insulin, or poor thyroid function, which is also explored in Puzzle Piece 6, The Thyroid). For an adrenally fatigued person, cortisol may be nice and low in the evenings or for some it starts to rise again, interfering with restorative sleep. Furthermore, if you don't go to bed before 10 p.m., an adrenally fatigued person will typically get a second wind, and it will be much harder for you to fall asleep if you're still up at midnight. The following graph illustrates this.

When morning cortisol falls low, it is likely that prior to this it was high (although not always), and body fat may have increased during this time. But just because it is low does not mean easy access to

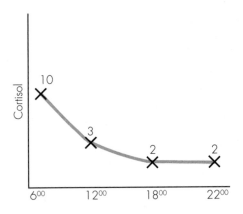

Figure 7: A typical cortisol profile of an adrenally fatigued person
Note particularly, the low waking cortisol and low midday reading.

body-fat burning, because of cortisol's relationship to insulin, as well as the catabolic effects of cortisol, described earlier.

Additionally, the fatigue you feel with this biochemical picture may make exercise the least appealing thing on the planet to you. You actually feel worse after exercise when you are adrenally fatigued, whereas exercise typically energizes us. Frustration mounts because you believe that exercising and eating less are the only solutions to weight loss, yet you can't bring yourself to do either despite every good intention. Every time you eat something sweet, you eat too much, or another month goes past without much movement. When you reflect on this, you feel guilty, you might say mean things to yourself—and you may silently lose hope. You now think, "Who cares?" whenever you feel like eating something that won't really nourish you, and the not-so-great eating continues, especially an excess consumption of carbohydrates as you desperately search for energy. Your clothes keep getting tighter and this just adds to your stress. The vicious cycle is self-perpetuating.

Humans were never designed to sustain long-term stress, and our individual bodies cope with it in different ways. For some, adrenalin remains the dominant stress hormone all of their lives, while others may flip over into what appears to be a more cortisol-dominant stress response. If the stress response doesn't truly switch off, there is the potential that the adrenals will eventually crash, and cortisol output is no longer optimum or elevated. It will be negligible. At its extreme, this is a condition called Addison's disease (and there may also be antibodies present), yet if a person's cortisol level is extremely low but still falls just inside the "normal" range, that person will be told that they are fine. They feel lousy but all the tests they have always come back "normal." They feel anything but normal, and people who know and love them will often comment that they are a shell of their former selves.

Cortisol can also be rather sinister in that it can interfere with your steroid (sex) hormone metabolism (explained in the next Puzzle Piece, Sex Hormones), your sleep patterns via its interference with melatonin, and also your mood via serotonin. Let's look at them.

The serotonin-melatonin seesaw

Is this your typical day? Healthy breakfast, mid-morning coffee, salad or sandwich for lunch... with probably something sweet to follow lunch, but other than that, you are quite proud of yourself when you reflect on your food consumption so far for the day. But I predict that many of you then fall into one of three categories. Do you:

1. Hit mid-afternoon and eat anything and everything in sight and then spend the rest of the day berating yourself after such a great start?

2. Get so busy during the afternoon that food does not enter your head until you arrive home and a glass of wine and possibly some cheese and crackers allows you to let out a sigh of relief that the day is winding down?

3. Or is it neither of the above and the free-for-all starts after dinner, when you find yourself standing in front of the

refrigerator or pantry saying to yourself, "I want something. I don't know what it is that I want but I want something. And maybe it's in here!"

Perhaps all three of these scenarios apply to you! Never fear, a new understanding is near.

All of these scenarios can have major emotional factors contributing to them. Emotional relationships to food are explored in Puzzle Piece 9, Emotions. However, on a physical level, options 1 and 2 are explored mostly as part of the insulin puzzle piece and are primarily about blood glucose. Option 3 describes "Captain Serotonin." Serotonin is our happy, calm, content hormone. It is the hormone that helps us feel like there is nothing for which we want in this world. It makes us very content with our lot in life. Melatonin is our sleep hormone and is responsible for sending us to, and keeping us, asleep. These hormones work antagonistically. That is, one goes up, the other goes down.

In our bodies we have what are called circadian rhythms, which govern a multitude of hormonal processes. These rhythms, coupled with fading sunlight, allow melatonin to rise, which, in turn, means serotonin must fall.

When a hormone that makes you feel happy, calm, and content decreases, it can create a noticeable sinking feeling, a distinct change in mood even though nothing in the external world has changed. Five minutes before, you felt fine, yet now there is this nagging feeling that you want something. There is a chance that a relatively lower level of serotonin as evening falls is partly why couples have conversations about "big ticket items" at this time of day. Our chemistry makes us feel like we want something and our brain tries to label what that might be. We usually don't find ourselves waking up and announcing that we absolutely must renovate the bathroom immediately! We keep those proclamations for evening. Serotonin has much to answer for.

Humans instinctively know that carbohydrate-rich foods promote serotonin production, which is partly why when the "I want something" syndrome hits, many people head for the pantry. They hope what they want is in there. Usually, though, guilt is all they find.

Mornings can also prove a challenge for someone in this pattern. Melatonin is destroyed by sunlight, which is partly why when we go outside and exercise in the morning we tend to feel great all day. The melatonin plummets when the retina of our eyes is exposed to light and, as a result, our serotonin surges. On a day where we get up and expose our eyes to sunlight, with that hormonal profile, we feel like we can cope with anything. The flip side, though, is not so appealing. If we've gone to bed after midnight, not slept well, or both, we may not want to rise with the sun, as we don't feel rested. If we just wander out of bed sometime during the morning, our melatonin slowly seeps away, and our serotonin slowly rises. On such a day, we feel like we need a few coffees to get ourselves going.

If this tale is ringing true for you, and the carb-fest in the evening feels out of control, the solution is not initially—or always—purely dietary.

Step one is to start getting up at the same time each morning and going outside and moving. Or at least open the curtains and recognize a new day has dawned, exposing your eyes to light. Welcome the day with tai chi, a walk, some yoga, or a stretch—whatever floats your boat. Commit to doing this for four weeks, every day, and observe if your evening carbohydrate cravings diminish. These rituals, combined with consuming more whole-food fats, can have a big impact on this biochemical picture. Your serotonin will love you for it.

How to support your adrenals

As you can see, cortisol plays many roles in our body, and optimal levels are essential for us to be able to access body fat to burn it, to feel content, have good energy, and keep inflammation and pain at bay. Is cortisol one of the factors you must address to solve your weight-loss puzzle?

How high your level of stress is and how you feel your body copes with it will influence the steps you take after reading this section. The first section of solutions is general, and I can confidently say that virtually everyone will benefit from applying them.

The herbs used for adrenal support are beautiful; however, it is best to check with a qualified medical herbalist to find out those that will meet your specific needs. I have made comments beside most of the herbs about their applications. If you have identified that you are adrenally fatigued and beyond exhausted on a daily basis, your adrenal support is listed separately on pages 64–65.

As you can already see, our perceptions play an enormous role in whether we are stressed or not. Sometimes it may be trauma in the past that takes a toll on the body. Even though you know in your mind you have dealt with it or moved on, your subconscious mind is still wrestling with it. Or stress can be from comparatively "little" things. It is as if you have an itch that somehow gets scratched by your beloved, your children, your boss, or by random people. Our bodies go through everything with us, and despite our minds consciously moving on; sometimes it is as if our bodies and biochemistry are stuck in the past. If this rings true for you, I suggest you read this entire book before you set about "solving" anything. After your first full read, return to each chapter, or puzzle piece, and construct your plan. Even more deeply, I hope that the messages on these pages will allow you to open yourself up to a new perspective on health, on food, on movement, on life, on feeling, on your beliefs, and, so importantly, on how safe you feel in this world. There are some wonderful methods through which you can help shift your body and your emotions when you feel like you have cognitively processed the living daylights out of your stress, yet it still remains a challenge or your weight is still stuck. These are listed below.

How your nervous system affects your health

At the heart of all of my strategies to support you adrenally is the desire for you to rest and to rest well, in a restorative and revitalizing way. Rest must follow action for us to have optimal health and excellent fat burning, and very few people these days truly rest, although we might believe we do. A part of our nervous system called the parasympathetic nervous system (PNS) is active when we truly rest. This is the "rest and repair" arm of our nervous system, but the opposite arm of the nervous system, the sympathetic nervous system (SNS), can dominate. This is described in more detail in a later chapter. For now, all you need to know is that if you do not lose weight from high-intensity exercise, it is likely that your SNS is dominant. If you do shift weight from this type of exercise, then your nervous system is likely to be well balanced. Both the PNS and the SNS are part of the autonomic nervous system (ANS). Understanding and supporting the nervous system is key to all aspects of wellbeing, as you will soon see in Puzzle Piece 8, The Nervous System.

The importance of breathing well

The other reason for this relatively brief section about the nervous system here is to make you aware of the cornerstone of all my adrenal support solutions and, just as importantly, explain *why* I will insist on this if you take nothing else away from this book: it has nothing to do with food, and it is absolutely free to everyone. It is breathing, and for some, it can be the key to shifting body chemistry from fat storage to fat burning. How is this possible?

The role of the ANS is to perceive the internal environment and, after processing the information in the central nervous system (CNS), regulate the function of your internal environment. The name "autonomic" implies that it is independent of the conscious mind. Think about a family of ducks and their newborn ducklings. Just like ducklings, the autonomic nervous system will always follow the leader, and the breath is the *only* part of the autonomic nervous system that can be controlled consciously. Your breath leads. Your body follows. The way you breathe offers your only access to your autonomic nervous system, and because we breathe 5,000 to 30,000 times a day—or 200 million to 500 million times in your lifetime—it has the potential to influence you positively or negatively in many ways.

Nothing communicates to every cell of your body that you are safe better than your breath. If you breathe in a shallow way, with short, sharp inhalations and exhalations, then you communicate to your body that your life is in danger. You have just learned about the cascade of hormonal events that follows such alarm and the role these hormones play in switching fat burning on or off. How you breathe is also a fast track to the symptoms of anxiety and, potentially, panic attacks, regardless of what led you to breathe in a shallow way in the first place, whether it was an event, a deadline, the perception of pressure and the consequent "need" to rush, or the lifetime habit of your nervous system. Long, slow breathing that moves your diaphragm communicates the opposite message to your body—that you are very safe. Nothing down regulates the production of fat-storage stress hormones more powerfully.

So, solution number one is to practice diaphragmatic breathing, making sure your tummy moves in and out as you breathe, as opposed to your upper chest. Schedule it at first until it becomes your new way of breathing (unless you literally do need to escape from danger such as slamming your foot on the brake, if another car suddenly drives out in front of you). Make appointments with yourself to breathe. If it is peaceful each morning while you boil the kettle for the first time that day (to make your hot water with lemon of course!), instead of racing around and doing 80 jobs while the kettle boils, stand in your kitchen and breathe diaphragmatically.

If you link breathing well to a daily routine, such as boiling the kettle or having a shower, it quickly becomes a habit. Do it numerous times over the course of your day. Book a meeting into your diary each afternoon at 3 p.m. If you work at a computer, have it pop up on the screen that it is time for your meeting with yourself to do 20 long, slow breaths. We keep appointments with other people, so be sure to keep the appointments you make with yourself. Take part in movement that facilitates a focus on the breath such as tai chi, qi gong, yoga, or walking quietly in nature. Pilates can also be useful, but I have found that it is highly dependent on your attitude while you are doing the session and also to some degree on the attitude of the instructor. This approach is partly about stilling the stories that we constantly hark on about in our mind.

The importance of laughter

Another free and powerful tool is laughter. If we see life as tough, full of hard work, pain, and drudgery, it will be precisely that. Humans have the ability to see only their perspective in the world, rather than the world as it truly is. We see the world through filters, yet we don't know they are there. I am not denying that life can be tough at times or that being honest with ourselves if we do feel down and out about life is not a good thing. The problem comes when we see the world this way and believe that it will never be any different. For then it won't be.

Think about it. A belief in the permanence of doom is dangerous for every hormonal signal in your body. Do your absolute best to shift your thinking to see life as an adventure, a journey and a gift, full of opportunity, a process through which we can contribute. Too many people are out of touch with how privileged their lives are given that all of their basic needs are met, as for too many people across the globe this is still not the case. Some of the greatest, most moving stories I have ever heard have involved someone turning a horrific hardship into their greatest opportunity. Keep this in mind.

Signs stress hormone production and/or the adrenals need support

- You feel stressed regularly and like you are on red alert

- You gained weight during or after a stressful period; you may have lost weight initially during the stress, but then regained that weight plus more

- Body fat has increased around your middle and the back of your arms, and you have grown what I lovingly refer to as a "back verandah"

- You crave sugar

- You love coffee and energy drinks—anything that contains caffeine

- You startle (jump) easily

- You don't sleep well

- You often wake up feeling unrefreshed

- You sometimes wake up feeling like you've been hit by a bus

- You feel better if you can sleep until 8 or 9 a.m., rather than arising between 5 and 7 a.m. Many of you won't have been able to assess this as you don't have a choice about what time you get up

- If you don't go to sleep by 10 p.m., you get a second wind and end up staying awake until at least 1 a.m.

- You regularly feel tired but wired

- You retain fluid

- Your face looks "puffy" or swollen at times (and other causes have been ruled out)

- You are a worrier; you don't relax easily

- You are a "control freak"

- Your body feels heavy and achy at times, even though you don't have a medical condition that warrants this

- Your blood pressure is high

- Your blood pressure is low or at the low end of normal

- You get dizzy easily, but particularly when you go from sitting to standing quickly

- You feel anxious easily

- You tend to experience low moods with no known other cause

- Your breathing tends to be shallow and quite fast

- You experience "air hunger" (and other causes have been ruled out)

- You struggle to say "No"

- You laugh less than you used to

- You feel like everything is urgent.

STRESS HORMONES SOLUTIONS

Just as important, if not the *most* important aspect of supporting adrenal function for a balanced and appropriate stress hormone response, is the application of the emotional health strategies (explored further in Puzzle Piece 9, Emotions) as well as conscious breathing. I know breathing sounds too simple to make a difference but diaphragmatic breathing (making your tummy move in and out as you breathe, as opposed to your upper chest) can literally change your life. And I don't say that lightly.

- Practice restorative yoga, Pilates, tai chi, or qigong a minimum of twice a week for four weeks. Develop a daily practice for outstanding results. My favorite is a practice known as Stillness Through Movement. Commit to a breath-focused practice.

- Spend five minutes daily focusing on and giving voice to all the aspects of your life for which you are grateful; you can't be stressed when you feel grateful.

- With the guidance of an herbalist, take some adrenal support herbs. Not all herbal medicine is created equal, however, so you want to ensure the brand you take is reputable. Check that it has been tested by a high-level quality-control system and that the active ingredients said to be in the product are indeed present, as well as no contaminants. Herbal medicine can be taken in a liquid tincture form or as tablets. The majority of the following adrenal herbs are adaptogens, meaning they help the body adapt to stress by fine-tuning the stress response. They include:

  > Withania for the worriers

  > Rhodiola for the drama queens or occasionally for the worriers

  > Siberian ginseng for the fatigued feminine

  > Panex ginseng for the utterly fatigued (short-term use only)

  > Licorice, especially if your blood pressure is on the low end of normal

  > Dandelion leaves, especially if you retain fluid

  > The adrenals also love vitamins B and C, and for adrenal support I usually supplement both: the Bs in the form of a multivitamin or a straight B-complex, plus 4–5g per day of vitamin C, preferably in powdered form with added calcium and magnesium, with the doses split over the day. If you are on an oral contraceptive pill, stick to 2g of vitamin C per day.

Adrenal fatigue supplementation

For people with deep, deep fatigue, I almost always use the following herbal tonic that contains:

- Panex ginseng

- Licorice

- Dandelion leaves

- Astragalus

- One other herb depending on what else is going on for the individual (a liver herb or a reproductive herb are typical)

I will also sometimes use a range of supplements specifically designed for people with adrenal fatigue. I usually suggest they trial them for three months and, when combined with the lifestyle changes outlined above (such as restorative practices and breath work), many have their energy and vitality return to great levels.

The restorative power of good food

Although I often recommend supplements of herbs and/or nutrients for adrenal fatigue, never underestimate the healing and restorative power of food the way it comes in nature. Taking supplements is not a reason to eat a poor-quality, low-nutrient diet. I simply recommend supplements where appropriate and especially to assist in the restoration of health. There is no pill that can make up for a lousy way of eating.

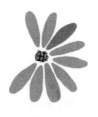

Puzzle Piece 3
Sex Hormones

Sex hormones can be delicious substances that give you energy and vitality, yet they can also wreak havoc in your life. When it comes to fat burning, beautiful skin, mental clarity, a sense of calm, the ability to be patient and not make mountains out of molehills, as well as fertility, very few substances in our body impact us more than our sex hormones.

The main sex hormones we will cover in this puzzle piece are estrogen and progesterone, with a particular focus on their role in body shape, size, and fat burning.

Can estrogen make you fat?

Estrogen is a feminine hormone (although men naturally make it in small amounts), and it plays numerous important roles in the human body, including those associated with reproduction, promoting new bone growth, and supporting cardiovascular health. The challenge with estrogen, however, occurs when there is too much of it compared to other hormones, progesterone in particular. Estrogen can also pose a problem if there is too much of one type of estrogen compared to other types of estrogen.

The ovaries of menstruating females make estrogen, and small amounts are produced by fat cells and the adrenal glands. At menopause, ovarian production of hormones ceases.

The role of estrogen in the female body from a reproductive perspective is to lay down the lining of the uterus, which it does between days one and 14 of a typical 28-day reproductive cycle, with day one of the cycle being the first day of menstruation. Estrogen lays the lining of the uterus down over these first 14 days to prepare the female body for conception, if it takes place. Estrogen prepares a menstruating female to fall pregnant every single month of her life, whether she wants to or not! Remember, our bodies are completely geared for survival, and perpetuation of the human species is an enormous part of that survival process.

As a result of the biological imperative to conceive each month, estrogen ensures there is adequate body fat, as most females will not know immediately that they have fallen pregnant. In the event that the woman is a stick figure without much body fat, it is possible that a brand new fetus may not survive. To prevent this, estrogen signals fat to be laid down in specific areas, broadening the hips for example, to better serve the childbirth process.

Estrogen is the hormone that makes female breasts bud at the first signs of puberty; it also broadens the hips, and gives us our curves. It lays down fat on a woman's hips, bottom, and thighs, and is typically responsible for making the lower half of a female body broader than the top half. Estrogen also, unfortunately, promotes fluid retention when it is in excess.

Fluid retention

I am convinced that many women "feel" fat when really they are either bloated or retaining fluid. I have never once weighed a client and I don't encourage anyone else to get on the scales either. I avoid "weigh ins" for many reasons, but one certainly is that hormone levels fluctuate over the month and can increase the amount of fluid being retained until the hormones return to balance. Besides, when you weigh yourself, remember that all you are really doing is weighing your self-esteem. I have met thousands of women who can gain 7lb (3kg) in a day, and to say that this messes with their mind is an understatement. If you get on the scales in the morning and weigh 143lb, and, by the evening, you weigh 150lb, especially if you have eaten well and done some exercise that day and even if you *haven't* eaten perfectly or exercised that day, it's easy to feel incredibly disheartened and wonder how on earth this could possibly happen.

Remember this: *It is not physically possible* to gain 7lb (3kg) of body fat in a single day. The only possible cause is fluid retention. Yet even though the logical part of the female mind will know this, seeing three extra kilos on the scales over the course of just a day, or even a week, will make most women, no matter how logical, feel fat, flat, and lousy. As an aside, are you more likely to make good food choices when you feel flat? Are you likely to want to be intimate with your partner when you feel fleshy and puffy? Usually not and then you (and they) feel worse.

There can be numerous factors behind fluid retention, too many to go into in detail here, but in a nutshell, fluid retention can be driven by poor lymphatic flow, mineral deficiencies and imbalances, poor thyroid function, excess stress hormone production, and poor progesterone production. From an energetic medicine perspective, think about who or what are you holding on to that no longer serves you? Perhaps it is a belief that you don't need anymore, and your body is simply trying to wake you up to this and get you to change. So many of us fear change, whether we realize it or not.

Estrogen can be a likely culprit when it comes to fluid in excess. It can also drive headaches, including migraines, increase blood clotting, decrease libido, and interfere with thyroid hormone production... big health consequences all due to too much of one little hormone.

What role does progesterone play?

Progesterone also plays a variety of roles in the human body. From a reproductive perspective, its job is to hold in place the lining of the uterus that estrogen has laid down between days one and 14 of your cycle. If your body detects that a conception has taken place, the lining of the uterus needs to be maintained and thickened, rather than shed. As a result, progesterone levels begin to rise. If there is no conception, the lining of the uterus is not needed, and progesterone levels fall away, which initiates menstruation. When health is optimal, progesterone is the dominant sex hormone from just after mid-cycle onward until menstruation.

Biologically, progesterone plays numerous other roles, all pivotal to the *Accidentally Overweight* message. Progesterone is a powerful antianxiety agent, an antidepressant and a diuretic, and it is essential if you are to access fat to utilize it for energy. Without the right amounts you will predominantly utilize glucose as your major fuel—not body fat—which may also lead to breaking your muscles down for additional energy, rather than burning fat.

The relationship between sex hormones and stress hormones is fascinating and powerful, and it's where a great proportion of the physical, biochemical approach of *Accidentally Overweight* is focused. And this is because the majority of women who attend my weekend events get very positive changes in their body and their health when we address this.

The relationship between stress and sex hormones

Estrogen is the dominant sex hormone between days one and 14 of the menstrual cycle. As described earlier, its job is to lay down the lining of the uterus and make sure there is enough body fat to support the early stages of conception, if this occurs. For the first half of the menstrual cycle, a relatively small amount of progesterone is made by the adrenal glands. For the sake of this description, let's call the amount two units. Remember, the reproductive role of progesterone is to hold the lining of the uterus in place, with the additional biological functions of it being an antianxiety agent, antidepressant, diuretic, and a support to using body fat as a fuel.

However, as you now understand from the previous chapter, your adrenal glands are also where you make your stress hormones, namely adrenalin and cortisol. Adrenalin communicates to every cell of your body that your life is being threatened, even though all you may have done is shown up at work and had an unexpected deadline thrown at you, or perhaps you had an argument with your beloved and he spoke to you inappropriately because he was feeling like a failure at the time. Men usually don't behave well when they subconsciously access failure as an emotion, while women typically behave in a way they (or those around them) don't like when they feel rejected. This does not excuse poor behavior, but rather offers an explanation to promote understanding.

When you are internally rattled, cortisol communicates to every cell of your body that there is no food left in the world and, as a result, it wants your body to break muscle down and store fat. Even though food is, in fact, abundant for you, and your cortisol production is likely to be coming from the areas of your life about which you feel uncertain, such as relationships, finances, or even what others might think of you, your body thinks there must be a flood, famine, or a war, as this was the only long-term stress humans historically experienced.

Since your body links progesterone to fertility, if your body's perception is that your life is in danger and that there is no food left in the world, the last thing it wants is for a woman is to conceive, so it shuts down adrenal progesterone production. Estrogen and cortisol, both signaling fat storage, remain, while you've lost the counterbalancing hormone that helps use fat as a fuel and also helps gets rid of excess fluid!

I believe this situation alone is a modern-day, monumental shift in female chemistry, and it can wreak havoc on a woman's emotional and physical wellbeing. A female can go from feeling happy, healthy, balanced, and energized, with great clarity of mind and an even mood, to having a foggy brain and feeling utterly exhausted. Physically she may feel puffy, heavy, bloated and full of fluid, with a sense that her clothes are getting tighter by the minute. And that is just the first half of the cycle!

A menstruating female ovulates around day 14 of her cycle, and there are numerous hormonal changes that occur to drive ovulation. Once the egg has been released from the ovary, a crater remains on the surface of the ovary where the egg popped out. This crater is called the corpus luteum, and it's where the bulk of a woman's progesterone is made. Progesterone is designed to peak on day 21 of a 28-day cycle at around 25 to 40 units. If conception takes place, then progesterone levels need to climb to continue to hold the lining of the uterus in place. Once the placenta has formed by week 12 of gestation, progesterone levels climb to around 300 to 400 units. Pregnancy is the time when a woman has the highest level of circulating progesterone in her lifetime. Once a woman has birthed, and passed the placenta, however, her progesterone level plunges from 350 to zero! It is fortunate that birth brings on some other feel-good hormones, although they tend to be more short-lived, and are impacted on by many environmental and emotional factors.

Historically, babies were welcomed into extended families and communities. Today, a more common scenario (not the only scenario) is a hospital birth followed by a new mother at home alone with her newborn during the day while her partner must continue to work to pay the bills. If there are challenges in their relationship or challenges caused by the demands of other children, financial stress, an ill newborn or simply one who won't sleep, the new home environment with baby can be highly stressful. Another stressful scenario I've heard described thousands of times is one where a new mum has made what she thought would be a welcome transition (temporarily or permanently) from a corporate career to staying at home with her baby, but is now second-guessing her decision. The guilt and confusion around this scenario can be overwhelming and do not promote the restoration of adrenal progesterone levels, as the body is so busy making stress hormones that it is not "safe" for the new mum to make the fertility-linked progesterone. Remember, progesterone is one of the most powerful antianxiety and antidepressant substances the body makes.

On the other hand, if mum and baby do have support, and the new mum doesn't feel she is alone with her precious new bundle, whether this is simply due to the mother's beliefs, attitudes, and perceptions, or her actual physical support from other people, then adrenal progesterone levels are far more likely to be restored, and her chemistry all the better for it.

If, on the other hand, conception does not take place during a menstrual cycle, then maintaining the lining of the uterus is no longer necessary, and progesterone levels fall, allowing a female to bleed. However, something that is so common today is what is known as "luteal phase insufficiency," where ovarian progesterone production is poor and a peak of 25 units in the second half of the cycle is not reached. Progesterone may be the dominant hormone from day 16 to day 18 of the cycle, but it falls away too soon (it is supposed to be dominant from around day 14/15 until around day 27), and estrogen becomes dominant leading into the menstrual bleed.

This estrogen dominance is the main biochemical basis of pre-menstrual syndrome (PMS), which causes grief for the woman as well as those around her! When PMS occurs it can be because estrogen is dominant for all but two or three days of a 28-day cycle, meaning that progesterone gets no time to rule the roost, and a woman misses out on all of its delicious stress-busting and fat-burning qualities.

What happens when estrogen is dominant?

The typical symptoms of low progesterone include:

- Premenstrual migraine

- PMS-like symptoms

- Irregular or excessively heavy periods

- Anxiety and nervousness

- A feeling like you can't get your breath past your heart

The typical symptoms of estrogen dominance (which usually also involves low progesterone—but not always) include:

- Irregular periods or excessive vaginal bleeding

- Bloating/fluid retention

- Breast swelling and/or tenderness

- Decreased libido

- Mood swings, most often irritability and depression

- Weight gain, especially around the abdomen and hips

- Cold hands and feet

- Headaches, particularly premenstrual

- Tendency to yellow-tinged skin.

This is the most common hormonal imbalance I see in menstruating women.

The impact of excess estrogen is not only having significant physical and emotional effects on too many adults, but children are now also being impacted at alarming rates. A growing percentage of girls are starting to menstruate as young as eight years of age, which is of enormous concern. The scope of this book, however, can't seek to "solve" this challenge but, for now, I merely want to highlight this "estrogen crisis" we currently face. The enormous excess of estrogen being made within the female body at earlier and earlier ages, often due to excess body fat (remember fat cells in girls, boys, women and men produce estrogen), combined with increased estrogen in our environment—predominantly from pesticides, herbicides and plastics (please never heat plastic of any kind; this means don't put it in the dishwasher)—appear to be affecting our endocrine (hormonal) systems in literally life-changing ways.

It is essential to discern whether a woman is suffering from symptoms of estrogen dominance due to excess estrogen or by significantly low progesterone levels, or both. Low progesterone typically signals that adrenal and/or ovarian production of progesterone is poor. This person may have optimal estrogen levels, yet they are challenged with their periods and/or their body fat due to low progesterone levels.

Another extremely common scenario is one of estrogen excess. This can come about through environmental exposures, such as those listed above, as well as those we may ingest through food or medications. Another significant basis for estrogen excess is estrogen recycling as a result of poor estrogen detoxification by the liver. I will explore this in detail later; however, in a nutshell, the liver decides whether to excrete or recycle estrogen.

The liver prioritizes what it needs to detoxify, and because the body makes estrogen itself, it is not a high priority to clear it from the body. The best way to imagine it is that a woman can have this month's estrogen circulating as well as last month's and even from numerous previous months. Even the best progesterone producer cannot keep up with so much estrogen. Regardless of where the estrogen comes from—internal or external sources—it is vital that it is detoxified and excreted efficiently, once it has done its job in the body.

An additional estrogen-dominant hormonal picture is a combination of both the descriptions above of poor progesterone production and recycled estrogen. If we took better care of our liver, this would be far less common in the Western world. As I love to say, these things have become common, but they are not normal. Women are not supposed to get PMS. Your period is supposed to just turn up. No fluid retention, no bloating, no food cravings, no mood swings… and if it doesn't just turn up, see it as your body asking you to do something differently: eat, drink, move, think, breathe, believe, or perceive in a new way.

I wrote the following article for breast cancer awareness month. The brief I was given was to write about what makes breasts healthy. Some of it repeats information I have included earlier, but I have shared it here to remind you how important these factors are.

Healthy breasts

When it comes to breast health, there is so much we now understand that contributes to the creation and maintenance of healthy breast tissue. Empowering women to take charge of this incredibly important aspect of their health is vital to the future of all women, and education must begin at a young age. Part of the challenge is distinguishing fact from fiction or fad, so let's explore what we know creates healthy breasts.

Hormones, stress, and the liver

Although the hormone estrogen does some wonderful things for our health, too much of it or too much of a particular type of estrogen has been linked to some breast cancers. What is important to explore, when it comes to our hormones, is, why is estrogen so much more of a problem now as opposed to a time in the not so distant past? Part of the explanation lies in the production of stress hormones, and part of the explanation

78

lies with the excretion of estrogen following liver detoxification of this substance.

When we are stressed, we make either, or both, of our two major stress hormones, namely adrenalin and cortisol. Adrenalin communicates to every cell of your body that your life is in danger, and cortisol tells your body that food is scarce. As a result, levels of another sex hormone called progesterone, which has been shown to be protective against breast cancer (except those that are progesterone receptor positive), fall through the floor as the body links progesterone to fertility. If the body believes that your life is in danger and that there is no more food left in the world, the last thing it wants for you is a pregnancy.

And so begins part of the problem with estrogen because it is dominant in comparison to progesterone. This situation may also arise from synthetic forms of estrogen, such as from the oral contraceptive pill (OCP) or hormone replacement therapy (HRT).

The second scenario to consider involves the excretion pathway of estrogen out of the body. Once a unit of estrogen has done its job for a specific time, it is transported to the liver where it has to be transformed so that it can be excreted. There are two phases to this detoxification process. Over the years, the workload of the liver in its second stage of this cleaning process can get clogged, just like traffic on a motorway. Where once substances flew through the liver at 100 mph, they now crawl through at 20 mph. When this process becomes terribly overloaded from years of too much alcohol, caffeine, refined sugars, trans fats, synthetic substances, or the byproducts of bowel congestion (a tendency to constipation), the estrogen will undergo its first stage of change, but there is no room on the second stage highway. So the estrogen is released by the liver back into the blood stream and recycled. Your body is then faced with the new estrogen it continues to make from your ovaries (if you are still menstruating) and your fat cells, as well as the recycled form. It is this recycled form of estrogen that has been found to be up to 400 times higher in women with estrogen-sensitive breast cancer.

Looking after your precious liver is one of the best steps you can take to ensure your breast tissue remains healthy. Sadly, many women regularly over consume alcohol, and it is this regular overconsumption that has been undeniably linked to the development of cystic breast tissue and breast cancers. We have to get real about how much we are drinking. Heart organizations around the world suggest that two standard drinks per day (equivalent of two 3½oz/100ml glasses of wine) with two days off each week are acceptable. Cancer research suggests, however, that if you have a family history of breast cancer, there is no safe level of alcohol consumption. That is a massive statement. If alcohol is something you enjoy, don't drink it daily. Save it for special occasions. Sparkling water with fresh lemon or lime served in a glass you like can be a great alternative.

Caffeine—coffee in particular—has also been found to play a role in the creation of denser, cystic breast tissue. On the other hand, green tea has consistently been shown in numerous studies to be protective against many types of cancers, breast cancer included. Most people are astounded at the changes in their breasts when they take a break from coffee and alcohol.

As a woman living in the same world as all of you, a world with plenty of alcohol and caffeine on offer, I challenge you to take a break from these substances no matter how much you love or depend on them. Do it for one week, one little week out of your big long life. If you find that easy, do it for two.

Or better still, omit them for one or two menstrual cycles and notice how different your breasts feel.

Diet and exercise

When it comes to the aspects of our diets that are essential for healthy breast tissue, vegetables and fruits head the list. All of the cruciferous vegetables (the brassica family) have potent anticancer properties. Broccoli, in particular, contains sulphoraphane, a compound that helps the body begin to eliminate carcinogenic substances from the body in as little as 10 days after it is included in the diet on a daily basis. It also keeps estrogen from binding to and stimulating the growth of breast cancer cells, a vital step in keeping breast tissue healthy. The great news, too, is that sulphoraphane survives cooking. Eat broccoli, people!

Eat fruits and vegetables that are also rich in beta-carotene. On average, women with breast cancer tend to have lower levels of beta-carotene in their blood, although researchers cannot say whether this is a cause or a result of the disease. A longitudinal study found higher biological exposure to carotenoids, indicated by higher average total plasma carotenoid concentration measured at multiple time-points during a seven-year follow-up period, was associated with greater likelihood of breast cancer-free survival in women who had been diagnosed and treated for early stage breast cancer.[6] The safest and most effective way of maintaining healthy levels of beta-carotene is to consume five or more servings of dark-green, yellow, or orange vegetables and citrus fruits daily. We must eat our vegetables every day. No excuses!

Make an effort to minimize your consumption of fried foods and charcoal-grilled meats. Also, there is evidence to suggest that reducing our consumption of animal foods and basing our diet mostly on plant-based foods is incredibly beneficial to breast health and the prevention of breast cancer.

There is a growing body of literature to suggest that insulin resistance is now a contributing factor in numerous cancers.[7] Insulin is a hormone that can behave like a growth factor. It encourages all cells to grow: fat cells, healthy normal cells, and cells that may be precancerous or cancerous. The best way to limit insulin production in the body is never to base a meal purely on carbohydrates. The only carbs humans traditionally ate were those from berries, legumes, pulses, and root vegetables. Today, we are faced with a barrage of highly processed foods, rich in refined sugars and refined starches. Limit your intake of these. Omit them if you can. We also tend to forget that most alcoholic drinks are packed with sugars.

Remember it is what you do every day that will have the most impact on your health, not what you do sometimes. It is not about going without; it is about getting real when it comes to what you, as a woman, already know to be true. You know better than anyone when you have too much of a particular substance in your diet… whether it is alcohol, coffee, or sugar. Make the changes you know you need to make now. You will give your breasts a great chance of remaining healthy in the process.

Last, move your body. The benefits of regular movement are well documented for many areas of our health, including a reduction in insulin levels and body fat, both of which, in excess, have been linked to unhealthy breast tissue.

Nutrients for healthy breasts

Most of us have heard about the importance of iodine for optimal thyroid function and in the prevention of goiter. What we hear very little about is how vital iodine is to breast *health. The breasts concentrate iodine as do the ovaries, and the protective effects of iodine on breast tissue and in the prevention of breast cancer have been postulated from epidemiologic evidence and described in animal models.*[8-10] *Use a good quality salt that contains iodine, add seaweeds to cooking, or take a supplement at the right dose for you, best guided by an experienced nutrition professional.*

Also of great consequence to breast health is our dietary intake and ratio of essential fatty acids. These are predominantly found in oily fish, flaxseeds, walnuts and pecans, evening primrose oil, and borage oil. It can be difficult to eat enough of these vital fats on a daily basis, so a good supplement combining at least (sustainable and mercury-free) fish or flax with evening primrose oils can be a great addition to your daily diet. Start with two capsules in the morning and two at night.

Another mineral that is essential for healthy breast tissue is magnesium and, coupled with selenium, these nutrients have been shown to reduce the incidences of new breast cancers. Green, leafy vegetables are high in magnesium, while Brazil nuts are rich in selenium. Eat them daily, or take a supplement.

Vitamin C is one of the most important nutrients when it comes to so many aspects of our health. The list of wonderful activities vitamin C performs in the body is almost endless. It helps keep the immune system responding appropriately to stimuli, and hastens white blood cell response times.

Vitamin B6 has also been extensively researched when it comes to breast health. Eggs are a good source, as are bananas and avocados.

Herbs for healthy breasts

Two of my most favorite herbs work on the adrenal glands. These are rhodiola and the ginseng family. Both herbs are considered to be adaptogens, which means they help the body adapt to stressors by fine-tuning the stress response. These herbs tend to have a calming effect on the nervous system, which in turn helps promote appropriate sex and stress hormone production rather than extremes.

Other herbs that have been shown to be useful in creating healthy breast tissue are those that promote liver detoxification and bile production and release from the gallbladder. Bile is essential for the appropriate excretion of any fat-soluble substances from the body, including cholesterol and estrogen. Useful herbs include St Mary's thistle, globe artichoke, bupleurum and schisandra.

Minimize exposure to…

The final thing you need to know about the creation and maintenance of healthy breast tissue involves the things that are best kept to a minimum wherever possible. Minimizing our exposure to growth factor-like substances, including insulin, may be an important aspect of maintaining healthy breast tissue. Dairy products naturally contain growth factors, since the milk is designed to grow an 90lb (40kg) baby calf into a nearly 2,000lb (900kg) adult cow.

The growth factors naturally present in milk and milk products drive this growth. Humans, however, aren't designed to grow at these rates. If milk must be consumed, sheep and goats are smaller animals so their milks tend to drive slower, smaller growth rates. Alternatively, nut milks contain no growth factors. For people with diabetes who need insulin, eating a diet that limits the need for insulin without, however, compromising blood glucose levels is important.

There is also a growing and very concerning body of evidence that points at the importance of minimizing our exposure to plastics and pesticides. They disrupt our endocrine (hormonal) systems and can mimic estrogen. Recent research out of the United States shows that a large percentage of girls aged eight have hit puberty, leading to longer estrogen production over their lifetime. Furthermore, fewer pregnancies also lead to relatively more time spent in estrogen-dominant states. Researchers suggest that poor diet, lack of exercise, high body fat, and exposure to plastics are the likely culprits for the earlier onset of menstruation. We can make a really big difference to our health and our children's health by getting these lifestyle factors on track.

• • • • • • • • • • • • • • • • • • • •

Reproductive system conditions

There are numerous reproductive conditions that involve poor progesterone production or estrogen dominance in some way. Polycystic ovarian syndrome (PCOS) and endometriosis are two frequently diagnosed, but quite different, conditions.

Polycystic ovarian syndrome

In PCOS, the eggs in the ovaries ripen on the surface of the ovary but are not released. They harden and form cysts (hence the name of the condition). As you now understand, to obtain optimal progesterone levels, ovulation is essential, since the corpus luteum makes the majority of your monthly progesterone.

Other hormones are also involved in PCOS. The pituitary gland, which sits at the base of the brain, makes luteinizing hormone (LH) and follicle stimulating hormone (FSH). Just prior to day 14 of a typical cycle, both hormones increase, but in PCOS both of these hormones from the pituitary gland tend to flat-line. Testosterone, the dominant male sex hormone, and other androgens, also tend to be elevated—slightly or significantly—in women with PCOS.

The LH and FSH hormonal profile of an ideal menstrual cycle is illustrated in figure 8 below while the profile of someone with PCOS is represented in figure 9.

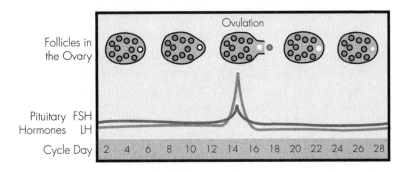

Figure 8: Ideal LH and FSH peaks generating ovulation
Both LH and FSH peak to drive ovulation.

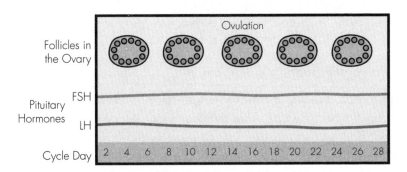

Figure 9: A typical PCOS LH and FSH profile
Both LH and FSH tend to flat-line in PCOS with LH
levels remaining consistently elevated.

Another hormone typically involved with PCOS is cortisol. It is usually high or very low (*see pages 47–51 and 55–57 in Puzzle*

Piece 2, Stress Hormones). In my clinical experience I have found that quite often, this is the first hormone that needs to be addressed before other hormonal patterns will shift.

Reproductive conditions and femininity

When it comes to challenges with the reproductive system or hormones, I find exploring subconscious beliefs and examining behaviors for each individual very useful. This is nowhere clearer than in PCOS. I often explain to my clients that there is nothing more feminine than our ovaries and in PCOS, it is as if the ovaries have gone deaf. The pituitary gland stops trying to alert the ovaries to release an egg, the most feminine process that goes on inside a woman. For the ovaries no longer to hear the call from the pituitary, there could be a very silent, unconscious belief from somewhere in this person's world that they have to behave like a man in order to receive appreciation, connection, or love. Somewhere in their past, more masculine behavior has been rewarded. Women are incredibly capable. They have shown they can match it with men in every arena. But there are types of work that, even today, are still more male-dominated. I have met countless women, working in these male-dominated industries in particular, whose hormonal profile has taken on a decidedly masculine appearance. These women, as I said, are incredibly capable. The problem, however, lies in their (usually subconscious) beliefs about how they have to be in order to perform and achieve. Most often, they do not even realize that they are thinking or behaving in this way until we explore what that looks like. Of course this isn't true for all women with PCOS and if this doesn't resonate then park it. I simply offer it here for you to explore, as it can be a missing part of the picture for many women with PCOS.

Our chemistry is ancient. What we ask of our body today is entirely different from what we asked of it even 50 years ago. On the one hand, it is truly remarkable what our body can do: Work 16-hour days sitting at a desk, constantly think up solutions to challenges presented during the day, meet deadlines, juggle phone calls, crises, and complaints, and hopefully also celebrate a few things along the way. And this is just the tip of the iceberg. On the other hand, we are so very far removed from the way humans have lived for 149,950 years that I believe the human body is rebelling, and one of the most obvious areas is women's reproductive health.

If this rings true for you, explore ways you can bring more feminine rituals into your life. What do you associate with femininity? If you need to be "masculine" at work, do it. Try instead to simply soften your thoughts when you're there. No one will know this is what you've done. Don't look at the work on your desk and tense up. Instead, notice the work on your desk and take a long slow breath that moves your belly when you inhale. Relax into it. Only you know you've done this. Your productivity and contribution will still be enormous and perhaps even more than what you found possible from a state of tension. Think about "creating" instead of "producing." In emotional medicine, the ovaries are the seats of creativity. Just that shift in language is more feminine.

When you come home, do something—at some stage in the evening—for you. Light a candle and notice the fragrance. Move your hips to music you love! Have a bath. Giggle with the children or at a comedy. Read a book if that appeals to you. Make a pot of herbal tea after dinner in a teapot you love, and turn it into an "occasion." Notice the design of the pot and cup, the fragrance, and how you feel taking care of yourself. Masculinity (not men, but masculine energy) would never do this. But a man embracing his feminine would, just to point out the difference.

Please understand, this not an antifeminist concept. Addressing the biochemistry of PCOS is of enormous importance to getting health results. I simply wanted to highlight the incredible benefit I have witnessed when women embrace their feminine essence in more areas of their lives and change the belief that they have to achieve to be loved. And feminine rituals are a beautiful place to start. I encourage all women with PCOS to explore what they perceive their fathers expected of them or whom they had to be to "earn" his love.

Endometriosis

Endometriosis is a condition where the tissue that is destined to line the uterus grows in areas outside the uterus. Just as the tissue that is laid down to line the uterus each month receives hormonal signals about when to shed, any uterine tissue that has been laid down elsewhere, such as around the fallopian tubes or attached to the bowel, also receives the same hormonal signals and this tissue also bleeds, which can be an intensely painful process. Furthermore, each area of tissue behaves like a little estrogen factory, adding to the already established estrogen-dominant hormonal picture.

Puberty

Some girls breeze through this time of transition without much change in their moods or their bodies, while, for others, anxiety or even a darkness can set in. Estrogen is the first female sex hormone to be made in any great quantity in a girl's body. As beautiful as estrogen can be as a hormone, it can wreak havoc when it is present in substantial amounts for the first time ever, in young female bodies that do not yet have sufficient progesterone being made to counterbalance its effects.

Prior to menstruation beginning, estrogen is being made, causing the breasts to bud and promoting the growth of pubic hair. It also begins to drive fat storage for all of the reasons outlined earlier. Some girls appear to be more "fleshy" for a time just prior to menarche, indicating estrogen is fulfilling its role.

Because progesterone is a powerful antianxiety agent and antidepressant, if it is slow to initiate, a girl who was once bouncy, bright, full of energy, and interested in things, can become flat in her moods and distant in her relationships. If her periods do begin and they are irregular and/or heavy and painful, to the extent she is unable cope with school or life in general, she will often be encouraged to go on the oral contraceptive pill. It is important to understand two things here. One is the way the contraceptive pills work and the second is the biochemical process that occurs at the onset of menstruation.

First, the pill is successful at preventing pregnancy because it shuts down the ovarian production of hormones, and hence ovulation. The number of women of all ages I meet who have no idea how this powerful medication works astounds me. I am neither pro-pill nor anti-pill; I simply want people to make informed choices. I will say it again. The pill shuts down ovarian production of hormones, and the body relies entirely on the synthetic version of hormones being supplied by the tablet. Substances in patented medications must be at least 10 percent different from the form the body naturally makes. They are not identical to the way the body makes it.

With the ovaries shut down, the adrenal production of progesterone becomes even more important, yet is unlikely to be optimal given what can be a stressful time around the onset of menstruation and, for some girls, the increase in body fat for the first time. Never never *ever* comment on an adolescent girl's changing shape and size by encouraging her to eat less. That stresses her more as she may feel like she is letting you down when she doesn't do it; it doesn't matter whether you are her parent, teacher, or friend. Explain that, for a while, hormones can change our shapes, and eating nutritious food and staying active are the most important things to do to stay healthy. With less stress, which may be due to her private perception of how her life is (which may gently be explored), her progesterone is more likely to kick in, and her body shape and size will sort itself out. Some areas that can be useful to explore in this situation are an adolescent female's perception of academic pressure and her perception of what it may mean to a family member if she "fails" (which may mean not coming out on top of her class in some cases). Exploring what her "friends" are saying at school can also prove insightful as her stress may be from the feeling that she doesn't fit in.

The second issue that needs to be explored is the biochemistry associated with the onset of menstruation. This is the first time in a girl's life that her pituitary gland sends signals to her ovaries. For approximately the first five years, the chemical messengers released by the pituitary follow a road to the ovaries that looks like a goat track, meaning that it is a path that sometimes reaches a destination (in this case the ovaries) and sometimes winds up heading off into no man's land. In other words, sometimes the pituitary signals miss their mark. After about five years, this pathway, if it has been allowed to become established, behaves like a five-lane highway. The route is clear, straight, and unhindered.

What I see, though, time and time again, are girls who have gone onto the pill to manage irregular or very heavy periods rather than for contraception, shortly after menstruation starts. And there are times when this is appropriate. If sport is a big issue or school is being missed due to severe period pain, then there may be scenarios when the use of the pill is appropriate, and I certainly do not want to elicit feelings of guilt in parents or daughters in this area. Just understand that the pill simply masks the truth and doesn't address why the periods are painful in the first place. If a girl stays on the pill long-term, the five-lane highway is never established. She will then come off the pill in adulthood wanting to have babies, but her pituitary has no history of communicating with her ovaries. It is a lot to ask our ovaries suddenly to wake up when we have suppressed their function for an extended period of time; for some women this is more than 20 years.

I cannot encourage you enough to get to the bottom of *why* the pain or the irregularity occurs in the first place. Before deciding about whether or not the pill is the best choice, explore other options and seek ways to change the hormonal imbalance that may be present, or if you can, at least give the pituitary-ovary pathway time to get established.

As far as moods are concerned, what breaks my heart is seeing a young woman start menstruating, with very heavy periods and some weight gain despite still eating well, disappear into her mind with her own private focus on sad thoughts. This can be the first time ever that a girl experiences a tendency to depression, and her family is often bereft and concerned at the change in their girl. The most common intervention in this situation is the prescription of the pill. But because the pill does not correct what is likely to be slow-starting, or insufficient, progesterone, the young woman's mood doesn't lift, despite her periods now being regulated (by the pill). So she is encouraged by well-meaning adults to take an anti-depressant. She is not even halfway through her teens, and she is on two of the most powerful medications in the Western world.

There are times when conventional medicine is lifesaving, and I am not suggesting it be avoided at all costs, especially not at the cost of precious human life. What I am encouraging, initially, is the balancing of estrogen and progesterone through natural methods with an experienced health professional. Counseling at the same time may also be incredibly beneficial to assist in dealing with the new darker thoughts that may have arisen. My holistic approach means also discussing any fears this young woman may have about her perception of what it means to be an adult woman. It can also be the first time she ever feels fleshy, puffy, or bloated, and, to a young mind influenced so heavily by popular magazines, it is easy to understand why she can think she is fat when all she is, is estrogen-dominant for the first time. As I said earlier, it is not physically possible to gain three kilos of fat in one day. It is most likely due to fluid and, given the diuretic action of progesterone, a deficiency of this vital hormone is one of the likely culprits of this young woman's fleshy and uncomfortable feelings.

Menopause

At its simplest level, menopause is the ceasing of the ovarian production of hormones. But production continues from the adrenal glands and body fat. However, as explained earlier, many women now make insufficient amounts of progesterone from their adrenals because of chronic stress. In my experience, this is such a powerful factor in whether a woman breezes through menopause with few or no debilitating symptoms, or whether the heat and the sleeplessness become overwhelming. If you are approaching menopause, I cannot encourage you enough to ensure your adrenal function is optimal. Apply the adrenal care techniques described earlier in this book, using breathing strategies and herbal support, combined with lifestyle changes where possible.

If you are post-menopausal, I also can't encourage you enough to address adrenal health and liver health (covered in the next chapter). Heat from the body can certainly be due to low estrogen levels or liver congestion. If I meet a client who has tried all sorts of natural estrogen therapies and used herbs that have an estrogenic action such as black cohosh, and they are still overwhelmingly hot and suffering debilitating hot flushes, I will treat their liver with the strategies outlined on pages 116–117 in Puzzle Piece 4, The Liver.

Remember that in traditional circles, menopause is a time when wisdom begins to flow constantly. Trust what you already know inside of you when it comes to your health. You innately know better than anyone else what is best for you. Seek guidance from health professionals, but apply what resonates for you.

Menstruation and menopause are feminine and very natural processes. They offer an incredible insight into a woman's general health, as well as a window into her inner world of unconscious thoughts and beliefs. These thoughts and beliefs drive so much of what we do and how we feel, and can be a barometer guiding her to remember what she was born knowing... that she is loveliness embodied.

Signs your sex hormones need support

- Your periods are heavy

- Your periods contain clots

- Your periods are painful

- You experience a heavy, dragging feeling as the menstrual blood passes

- Your breasts are swollen and/or tender in the lead up to menstruation

- You regularly experience headaches or migraines in the lead up to menstruation

- You experience mood swings in the lead up to menstruation— or at the same time each month, for example around ovulation—which swing anywhere from immense irritability to intense sadness, sometimes in the same hour, and often for no reason you can fathom!

- You experience PMS

- You've been diagnosed with a condition such as PCOS, endometriosis or fibroids

- Your skin breaks out with your cycle

- Your menstrual cycle is irregular

- You are experiencing a debilitating menopause

- Acne started at puberty and it hasn't resolved

- Weight gain occurred at puberty for the first time (can also be food-related and/or emotional)

- A tendency toward low moods occurred at puberty for the first time (can also be food-related and/or emotional)

- You retain fluid and this is worse in the lead up to menstruation

- You feel anxious in the lead up to menstruation

- You crave foods, often sweets, more so in the lead up to menstruation

- You feel a deep fatigue in the lead up to menstruation

- You are having challenges conceiving

- You have "unexplained infertility"

- Your bowel habits change (either to constipation or diarrhea) in the lead up to, or during, menstruation

- Your head feels "foggy" in the lead up to menstruation

- You take painkillers during menstruation

- Most months you have a day/s off due to menstruation challenges

- You feel like you can't get your breath past your heart (and down into your belly) in the lead up to menstruation

- You have pimples/congested skin/acne on your back or chest

- "Unexplained" weight gain, particularly around the abdomen and hips

- Cold hands and feet. This is worse in the lead up to menstruation

- Tendency toward yellow-tinged skin (which is not caused by other factors, such as a liver disease)

- You experience poor (or worse) sleep quality in the lead up to menstruation.

SEX HORMONES SOLUTIONS

For all the challenges discussed in this chapter, focus on the gifts of your feminine essence, while the following solutions give more specific advice.

For menstrual or reproductive system

- If you have any type of menstrual cycle or reproductive system challenges, take a four-week break from alcohol or, better still, take a break from it for two menstrual cycles. You'll see your PMS significantly decrease.

- If this solution is "impossible," decrease alcohol intake to two nights a week, and preferably drink less than half a bottle of wine. I meet so many women who drink a minimum of half a bottle of wine every night. We were never designed to drink in this way. Decrease it.

- Coffee can be another big-ticket item when it comes to PMS, via liver congestion. Consider swapping coffee for green tea for four weeks, and see how you feel.

For estrogen dominance (which can be confirmed with a saliva or a blood test)

- Products containing broccoli sprouts.

- Diindolylmethane (DIM), an extract of broccoli.

- Organic green drinks: powdered/ground green vegetables and grasses that you add to water. The reason juices and smoothies aren't listed here is that often people add too much fruit to them in an attempt to make them palatable. Good-quality, organic green powders offer concentrated sources of some key active ingredients that help support efficient liver detoxification, particularly estrogen metabolism.

- Products containing curcumin, turmeric, or beetroot can also assist.

Note: I am all for getting what we need from our food, but, in this case, you would need to eat about eight heads of broccoli a day to get the same therapeutic effect as one good-quality capsule (from a reputable, quality-assured brand) containing broccoli sprouts or similar.

Menopause strategies

- For hot flashes (flushes) consider whether the heat is coming from low estrogen, liver/gallbladder congestion, or both?

- For low estrogen, black cohosh and sage can be useful.

- For the liver/gallbladder, globe artichoke, St Mary's thistle, bupleurum, or schisandra are excellent.

- For adrenal support, rhodiola can be brilliant if you are also exhausted or Siberian ginseng or withania.

- For low blood pressure, licorice is excellent.

- Magnesium.

For PMS

You may experience one or a number of different PMS patterns at once, and find the following table describes the different types of PMS—the mechanisms involved and the potential treatments.

	SYMPTOMS	MECHANISM	POTENTIAL TREATMENT
PMT-1	Anxiety Nervous tension Irritability Mood swings Insomnia	Elevated estrogen Low progesterone High cortisol	Vitex Dong quai Vitamin B DIM
PMT-2	Water and sodium retention Abdominal bloating Weight gain Breast tenderness	Elevated aldosterone (fluid) Low dopamine	Dandelion leaves Vitamin B Vitex Rhodiola
PMT-3	Craving sugar Increased appetite Can't resist refined sugar, followed by palpitation and fatigue Dizziness, shakiness, headache	Low magnesium Deficiency of prostaglandin PGE1 (low in anti-inflammatory substances) Elevated insulin	Magnesium Essential fats; Udo's oil or fish oil or a flax oil and evening primrose oil combination Cinnamon
PMT-4	Period pain and clots	Elevated prostaglandin PGE2 (pro-inflammatory; increases inflammation in the body) Deficiency of anti-inflammatory substances Possible magnesium deficiency	Bupleurum if clots Dong quai Magnesium Essential fats, fish oil, flax oil if vegetarian

Puzzle Piece 4
The Liver

When it comes to fat burning, the liver packs a mighty punch. In conjunction with the gallbladder, it works endlessly to help us excrete fatty substances, including stored body fat. The best way to imagine the fat-burning power of the liver accurately is to picture a triangle shape on its side, and inside that triangle are billions and billions of little circles, each one of them a liver cell. Inside each liver cell is a mouse on a wheel running and running and running, and each turn of the billions of little wheels is contributing to driving your metabolism.

When we treat our liver unkindly, a circle (liver cell) can die. For a time, the liver can regenerate a dead cell, but, after a while, this is no longer possible, and a globule of fat will take up residence where once that fat-burning little "mouse" was working. When many fat globules take over the liver (known as "fatty liver"), our body-fat deposition pattern shifts. For the first time, people notice that they have a fat roll quite high up on their abdomen. For women, this is just below their bra line and, for men, just beneath their pectoral muscles. It can come and go, and sometimes there is a point right in the middle of your torso that is tender. I will always suggest ways to support your liver based on the presence of a fat roll in that position and gallbladder support based on that tender point.

It is not, however, only fat burning itself where the liver plays a role in body-fat management. The liver also guides other areas of metabolism, including cholesterol and estrogen, which are important to understand when it comes to health in general, as well as accessing fat to burn.

The nutrients you need for detoxification

The liver is the body's second largest organ after our skin (although if you count the endothelium—the thin layer of cells that line all of the blood vessels and lymphatic vessels—as an organ the liver is the third biggest organ). It sits just behind your right rib cage. Its primary role is detoxification, a concept surrounded by much confusion. Detoxification is a process that goes on inside us, all day every day, and is essentially a transformation process in which any substance that would be harmful to you, if it were to accumulate, is changed by the liver into a less harmful form, so it can then be excreted safely from your body and gone forever. The lifestyle choices we make influence how efficiently the liver is able to do its job.

There are technically three stages to the liver detoxification process; however, nothing is lost and it tends to be easier to understand if I simply explain it as a two-step process.

The two stages to the detoxification process are appropriately named phase 1 and phase 2 liver detoxification pathways. Figure 10 opposite illustrates the phases of detoxification. Both stages require certain nutrients to function, and dietary choices can influence how efficiently each phase is able to proceed.

For the first stage of detoxification, numerous nutrients, including B vitamins, are essential. Grains are one of the richest sources of B vitamins we have in the food supply, yet many people feel much better eating fewer, if any, of these foods. People decrease or cut grains out of their diets for varied reasons. Some first experienced rapid weight loss with the advent of the high-protein, very low-

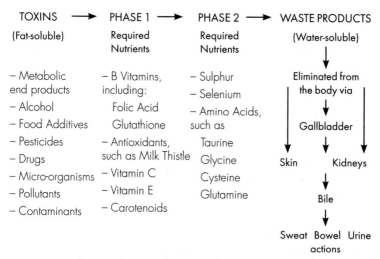

Figure 10: Detoxification Pathways in the Liver

carbohydrate diets, purported as the answer to all of our weight loss desires in the late 1990s—a repeat of the popular dietary concept from the 1970s. Some people simply started to notice that foods made from grains gave them reflux or made their tummy bloated and took action to change how they felt.

If grains feel good for you and energize you, then enjoy them in whole-food form. If they don't suit you, don't eat them. Your body knows best what works for you. Simply be aware that if you have a low intake of B vitamins, your phase 1 liver detoxification processes may not function optimally. It can be useful to take a supplement if you eat a low-carbohydrate diet or avoid or limit grains.

There is one road into the liver (the phase 1 pathway) and five pathways out of it (the phase 2 pathways). Just as for phase 1 reactions, phase 2 liver pathways also require certain nutrients to function, in particular, specific amino acids and sulfur.

Really think about this next statement: *What you eat becomes part of you.* The protein foods you eat are broken down into amino acids, and one of the things they go on to create is all of the cells of your immune system, which defends you from infection. Amino acids also go on to create the neurotransmitters in your brain that influence your mood and clarity of thought. They also build your muscles so that you can carry your groceries and children. It really does matter what we eat. Your food becomes part of you.

We obtain dietary sulfur from eggs, onions, garlic, and shallots, as well as the brassica family of vegetables, which includes broccoli, cabbage, kale, Brussels sprouts, and cauliflower. The liver makes enzymes that are responsible for the transformation of each substance, and the rate of production of these essential enzymes determines how quickly each substance is processed. If there are nutrient deficiencies, the amount of and that rate at which liver enzymes can be made, will be compromised. The load placed on the liver as a result of—for example—dietary choices, environmental factors, gut health, and estrogen metabolism also determines how quickly things move through the liver.

Liver loaders

There is a group of substances that I lovingly label "liver loaders." Can you guess what they are? They include:

- Alcohol

- Caffeine

- Trans fats

- Sugars, including fructose and sucrose (*see also the further explanation on page 159 of Puzzle Piece 7, Insulin*)

- Synthetic substances, such as pesticides, medications, skincare products, etc.

- Infection, for example viruses such as glandular fever (Epstein-Barr virus, mononucleosis, etc.)

When it comes to pesticides we are guinea pigs with regards to the long-term consumption of these substances. The reason your apple looks so perfect is because it has been sprayed to make it that way. We cannot see or taste the chemicals on its skin, but they are there. Pesticides have to be tested before they can be used on food for human consumption. However, they are often tested for such a short amount of time that I do not believe we can compare tests done over, say, a six-month period, to being exposed to these things over our entire lifetime. What also cannot be tested is what happens when all of the chemicals are mixed and then combined inside our bodies every day when we eat conventionally grown produce.

Fresh food the way it comes in nature is an incredibly important part of our diets, and I simply want to encourage you to choose organic produce whenever you can. Also, think about the way you eat the food. We peel a banana. It may have been sprayed, but how much gets through the skin? We actually don't know. But surely there would be less chemical residue in the flesh (inside) of a banana than on the skin. So perhaps choosing a conventionally grown banana is not too bad. Yet when it comes to an apple, we usually eat the whole fruit. So you would be better to choose an organic (or biodynamically grown) apple wherever possible.

Think about this. Organic food is the true cost of food. I once started and ran an organic café. Once a week, a local farmer delivered fresh greens picked that morning from his biodynamic farm. I always set aside some time on the day of his delivery to chat with him, as he always had wonderful tales to tell of life on his farm. One day, when I asked him how he was, his reply was along the lines of "not so good." When I enquired further, he went on to tell me that snails had invaded his broccoli patch virtually overnight. When I paused to consider this, I realized that, if they took hold, a portion of this man's meager livelihood would be lost. So I asked him how he deals with snails on his broccoli given that his farming principles do not involve spraying the patch to get rid of the invaders (which would have taken less than 30 minutes to do). My farmer friend went on to tell me that snails lose their "stick," their ability to suction on to things, in salty water. So he made up a bottle of salt and water, and he spent two days, crouched down on all fours, crawling between his broccoli plants, squirting saline water up under the fronds. Not only that, he didn't kill the snails but collected them in a bucket and fed them to the chickens "to keep them in the food chain," as he so delightfully put it.

Think about each of these scenarios. Spray in under 30 minutes versus crawling around on your haunches for two days. For me, that illustrates precisely why organic and biodynamic food costs more. It reflects the real cost of food, plus it has a greater nutritional value, not to mention what's left out. The more of us who choose it, the cheaper it will become. The more we demand organic and say no to pesticides, the more organics will have to be supplied. I know I'm on my soapbox, and I really do want to remain real and practical with the advice I offer. So, in simple terms, choose organic food whenever you can.

If organic food is unavailable in your area or it is too costly for you to buy, try this solution to remove pesticides. Pesticides tend to be fat-soluble and general washing to get rid of dirt and germs does not remove them. To clean food of both dirt and pesticides at the same time, fill your sink with three parts water to one part vinegar, and wash your fruits and vegetables. Then rinse them in fresh water, pat them dry, and store them for use. Do what is practical for you.

Another consideration, in the liver-loading department of synthetic substances, is the skincare we use. We're crazy if we think that we don't absorb things through our skin. You only have to look at the way nicotine patches work to realize that the skin is a quick and easy route to our bloodstream, carrying the blood that the liver will need to clean. There are plenty of wonderful skincare companies out there that do not use synthetic ingredients. Seek them out. I love to suggest to people that it would be good if they could eat their skincare!

It is not, however, just the things we consume or the things we put on our skin (exogenous liver loaders) that can place demands on the detoxification processes of the liver. Substances your body makes itself (endogenous liver loaders) also need to be transformed by the liver so they can then be excreted. These substances include:

- Cholesterol

- Steroid hormones such as estrogen

- Any shortfall in digestion/bowel congestion/irritable bowel syndrome (IBS).

I have met countless people who have not consumed much in the way of exogenous liver loaders, but they still have diabolical menstrual cycles or an ongoing challenge with IBS or constipation, and exhibit what I consider to be very distinct signs that their liver needs support. Passing clots while menstruating is a classic liver congestion sign (other symptoms are listed on page 116 of this chapter).

My point is, if your body thinks it is in your best interest to produce excessive amounts of cholesterol in the liver—often due to inflammation—or if your bowels have been the bane of your life for many years, it is likely that you would feel much better and your clothes would become looser if some liver support strategies were employed.

Cholesterol

Cholesterol is an extremely important substance. We only ever hear bad press about cholesterol; however, we would melt without it. It is the building block of all of our steroid (sex) hormones, including progesterone and testosterone. The process that cholesterol undergoes to form steroid hormones is illustrated in figure 11 following.

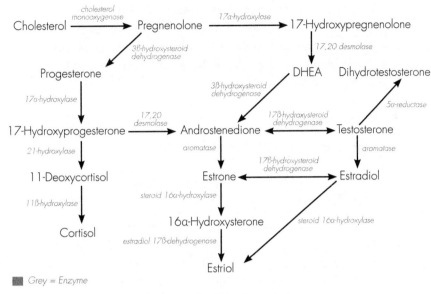

Figure 11: Cholesterol metabolism
The creation of steroid hormones from cholesterol.

The reason I've included the above biochemical diagram is to illustrate the way substances in the body flow on to create other substances. Cholesterol that the body makes, or that you obtain from your diet, does not always remain as cholesterol. In fact, you do not want too much cholesterol accumulating as cholesterol. You want it to turn into progesterone, testosterone, DHEA, and estrogen (all of the words in the diagram that begin with "est" are different forms of estrogen).

Your diet contributes to approximately 20 percent of the amount of cholesterol in your blood, while your liver creates the other 80 percent. Your liver makes cholesterol when it needs to protect itself and, in such situations, cholesterol behaves like an anti-inflammatory. What are some of the things that may inflame the liver and drive additional cholesterol production? We listed them above! Furthermore, with more and more people having digestive system challenges and with the increase in autoimmune diseases (remember that about 80 percent of the immune system lines the gastrointestinal tract) for some people, specific foods can also drive an inflammatory response. An experienced health professional can guide you with this, if it is part of your health picture.

One of the most successful ways to reduce your blood level of cholesterol is to take extra good care of your liver and deal with any inflammation in the body with a good-quality essential fatty acid supplement, outlined in the solutions on page 117 later in this chapter. Another mechanism involved in the accumulation of cholesterol is outlined below.

Based on the cholesterol metabolism flow chart shown in figure 11, healthy cholesterol metabolism is best imagined as a gently flowing stream. You want a small amount of cholesterol to remain in your blood as cholesterol, but you want the majority of the cholesterol to be converted into your steroid hormones. Men and women make all three of the major sex hormones—specifically testosterone, estrogen, and progesterone—they just make them in differing ratios, with men producing more testosterone and far less estrogen with some progesterone, while women make more estrogen and progesterone and less testosterone. You can see in figure 11 (opposite) how certain enzymes push the hormones one way or the other.

Sometimes over time, however, cholesterol can accumulate as cholesterol. To come back to the analogy of cholesterol metabolism being like a flowing stream, it is as if a dam wall gets built across the flow and, instead of cholesterol being converted into sex hormones, it accumulates in the blood as cholesterol. There are two problems here.

1. Too much blood cholesterol may pose a health problem (although the jury is out on whether this is actually true with regard to heart disease)

2. Lower levels of sex hormones are being produced. Since your steroid (sex) hormones make you feel vital and alive, they play

an enormous role in whether you bounce (or stagger) out of bed each morning. When you have optimal levels of, and balanced, sex hormones, you feel amazing.

For cholesterol to be converted into sex hormones, you must have optimal zinc levels, and essential fatty acids are also important. Our best sources of the omega 3 fats are the oils in fish, flaxseeds (linseeds), walnuts, and pecans, while evening primrose oil and borage oil are good sources of the omega 6 type. The richest food source of zinc is oysters. Beef and lamb also contain some, and vegetable sources include seeds, such as sunflower seeds and pumpkin seeds. As far as amounts go, however, oysters contain (on average) 70mg of zinc per 100g, whereas beef, the next best source of zinc, contains only 4mg per 100g. Lamb has on average 2.9mg of zinc per 100g; seeds have around 0.9mg of zinc per 100g. In the not so distant past, we obtained consistent amounts of zinc from our plants foods. But food is only as good as the quality of the soil, and if a nutrient is not in the soil, then it can't be in our food! Most soil in the Western world is deficient in zinc these days unless it has been organically or, better still, from a zinc perspective, biodynamically farmed.

Each adult needs a minimum of 15mg of zinc per day, just so the body can perform its basic functions. That is potentially not even enough for optimal health. So from where on earth are we getting our zinc? The answer is, many of us are not. Some studies have suggested that approximately up to 70 percent of people living in Western countries are deficient in zinc, even though it is a mineral that is not only essential for keeping cholesterol levels in check and producing optimal amounts of sex hormones, but it is also vital for our skin and wound healing, as well as digestion and immune function. Zinc is a mighty little mineral.

Excretion of cholesterol and estrogen

The second part of this biochemical picture about cholesterol metabolism and liver health involves the excretion of cholesterol. The same mechanism also applies to estrogen—so for any female who read the previous puzzle piece and identified estrogen dominance in her life, this is incredibly important.

When a liver loader, either exogenous or endogenous, arrives at the front door of the liver, it has arrived to be changed. Alcohol, in particular, must be changed as a priority, since the human body is unable to excrete it. I do not make the following statement lightly; it is simply a fact. *Alcohol is a poison to the human body.* We cannot excrete it. To do so it must be changed into acetaldehyde. Acetaldehyde is the substance that can accumulate and cause a headache/hangover the day after excessive imbibing.

So when any of the liver loaders (in this case, let's remain focused on cholesterol) arrive at the front door of the liver, they undergo the first stage of change (phase 1 liver detoxification). Between the front door and the middle of the liver, cholesterol is still cholesterol, although it has been slightly changed. This slightly changed cholesterol then wants to go down one of the five phase 2 detoxification pathways and, once it has done that, it has been slightly changed again, and it is this substance that can then be excreted and gone from your body forever.

Health problems can arise, however, when the traffic on the phase 2 pathways gets jammed like traffic on a highway. After years of routine consumption of liver loaders, and hormonal or bowel problems, the roads out of the liver can become congested. Conventional blood tests for liver function do not show this. The liver takes years of battering before conventional blood tests reflect the congestion that led to them becoming elevated in the first place. When the traffic is jammed, the cholesterol (or estrogen) undergoes its first stage of change and arrives in the middle of the liver, ready to go down its appropriate path for the second stage of the transformation it must undergo before it can be excreted. If the phase 2 pathways are clogged, the cholesterol (or estrogen) sitting in the middle of the liver has nowhere to go, but it cannot remain waiting in the middle of the liver, as there is more garbage constantly coming through the front door. When this happens, the best way to imagine it is that the liver has a trap door, and it releases the cholesterol (or estrogen) back into the blood and the recycling of that substance begins. It is the recycling of these substances, not the substances themselves, that is potentially harmful to human health. What organ can we take much better care of if we want to stop this recycling from happening? Our precious liver.

On another note, it is the recycled form of estrogen that is of such concern for women regarding the risk of developing numerous reproductive cancers. Estrogen is a beautiful hormone in the right amount and with the right types of estrogen being dominant. Too much total estrogen or too much of the wrong type are the problems, because of the estrogen itself and also because progesterone production can never match it. Our livers need more love and less of a load.

Antioxidant defense mechanisms

The other way the body detoxifies (other than by phases 1 and 2 detoxification pathways) is through our antioxidant defense mechanisms. This is a superb aspect of our chemistry. Humans stay alive through a process called "respiration," meaning that we breathe in oxygen, and we exhale carbon dioxide. If you could see oxygen in space, it is two Os (two oxygen molecules) stuck together. Figure 12 below illustrates what I am about to describe.

$$O_2$$
$$O = O$$
$$O$$
$$A/O$$
$$O = O$$
$$O_2$$

Figure 12: Free radical protection from antioxidants
The oxygen donation of antioxidants.

When we breathe, oxygen splits apart, forming two single oxygen molecules. These are known as free radicals, and they are angry little critters, as they have lost their buddy. They have the potential to damage your tissues. One of the main ways the body defends itself from damage by a free radical is through the consumption of antioxidants. Antioxidant-rich foods are our colored plant foods. Blueberries, green tea, red wine, and chocolate are rich in antioxidants and the most common antioxidant-rich foods called out at my live events when I ask the audience for ideas! It is the skins and seeds of red grapes that are especially high in antioxidants, so grape juice is just as powerful as red wine (from an antioxidant perspective!). If you could imagine a large platter covered in beautiful, brightly colored fresh produce, that platter would pack an antioxidant punch, and we want to obtain the majority of our antioxidants from our plant foods.

The way it works is that the antioxidant donates one of its oxygen molecules back to the single guy (free radical) and they pair up. The oxygen is then as happy as a duck again; it has its buddy back and will no longer damage your tissues. Isn't that magical?

To understand one powerful way free radicals can damage our tissues is to imagine a blood vessel leading to your heart. A free radical zips about through the blood and suddenly does a dive bomb and makes an indentation in the wall of the vessel. It resembles the divot in the grass beneath a golf swing that has taken too much soil with it. The damaged vessel sends out a cry for help, and, in this case, cholesterol—that up until now has been floating along in your bloodstream—wants to be the hero.

Cholesterol behaves like a Band Aid in this situation, coming along and sticking itself over the top of the injured site. It then sends out a message to all of its cholesterol friends to join the party, and they too come and stick themselves over the top of the first cholesterol globule that arrived. The cholesterol piles up, and then it oxidizes and hardens. This is one form of atherosclerosis or plaque, and it narrows the interior of the arteries—garbage can also accumulate inside the walls of blood vessels. Where once the blood could flow through a wide, open vessel, it now has a very narrow, restricted path to follow. Your blood is the only way for oxygen and nutrients to get around your body. Your heart is a muscle, and it needs both oxygen and nutrients to survive. If it is starved of either of these for long enough, this is one way we can go on to have a heart attack.

The good news, though, is that this condition is reversible. The hardened, built-up cholesterol is LDL cholesterol, which is why it is commonly known as "bad" cholesterol. "Good" cholesterol (HDL cholesterol) comes along and unsticks each globule of cholesterol and carries it off. Where to? You guessed it… the liver. It arrives at the front door of the liver to undergo its detoxification process and, when the liver is functioning well, the cholesterol is processed, excreted, and gone forever. However, if the liver is loaded up with substances with higher priority up the detox order than boring old, home-made cholesterol (in other words most other substances entering the liver), then the cholesterol reaches the midpoint of the liver, is released too soon, and gets reabsorbed. And that is one major way our blood cholesterol goes up and up and up. Cholesterol can also be elevated when thyroid function is poor.

I don't say this to blow my own trumpet but simply to demonstrate the power of outstanding liver function: in the 17 years I have been working with patients, there is not one person whose blood cholesterol I haven't lowered back into the normal range, simply by helping them to take better care of their liver. Not one. It doesn't matter if cholesterol levels are through the roof, or only slightly elevated and the GP/MD wants it back into the "normal" range, the body responds. And even more miraculously for the majority of people this occurs in less than eight weeks. No medications, just appropriate dietary change and liver support. Given the critical role cholesterol plays in metabolism, I am not overtly concerned with its elevation in the blood. What matters to me is a *change* in the level for an individual, as something has caused this. I see elevated blood cholesterol as a reflection of biochemical processes that need attention, such as the phase 2 liver detoxification pathways. The cholesterol itself is unlikely to be a problem; it is what has led to its elevation that must be addressed.

The following is an article I wrote about alcohol that was published in a January issue of a magazine.

Alcohol

As the festive season draws to a close, the effects of too much alcohol may still be silently, or loudly, reverberating. Whether it is increased body fat or cellulite, less energy and vitality, worse bouts of PMS or mood fluctuations... or perhaps your get up and go has got up and left. As fun as it can be at the time, alcohol can rob you of your clarity and purpose. And so January often sees us making big statements about our health, alcohol reduction, or avoidance. Some wait until February to take a break, as they've worked out it has fewer days! I know others who do Oct-sober in October.

We drink for wide and varied reasons. For some, it is the way they socialize, or the way they wind down from the day. Some use alcohol to distract themselves from thoughts and feelings they'd rather avoid. It can be a way that people cope. Regardless of the reason, many of us over-drink without even realizing it.

A standard drink is 100g of alcohol in whatever form that comes. In New Zealand and Australia 100g of alcohol is a 330ml bottle of 4 percent beer, a 30ml nip of spirits, 170ml of champagne, and it is a measly 100ml of wine—about four swallows! Next time you pour yourself a glass of wine, measure it, and see what your natural pour is. For most, it is considerably more than 100ml, and, as a result, many of us are over-drinking without even realizing.

The current recommendations provided by heart organizations say that for women, no more than two standard drinks per day with two alcohol-free days (AFDs) per week is okay, while for men, three standard drinks per day and two alcohol-free days is acceptable.

We have long heard the heart-health benefits of red wine publicly sung, and somehow it justifies to too many that drinking is OK—you tell yourself you are clearly looking after your heart. Also consider the American Cancer Society's position statement on alcohol. It is very powerful and they "recommend" even less is consumed. Studies have suggested that if you have a family history of cancer there is no safe level of alcohol for you to consume.

I'm not suggesting you don't drink alcohol, if you like it. Alcohol consumption can be immensely pleasurable for those who partake. I simply want to appeal to you to get honest with yourself about how alcohol affects you. You know in your heart if you drink too much and when it is impacting negatively on your health. Alcohol can affect the way we relate to those we love the most in the world, and of course it affects how you feel about yourself. It has a depressant action on the human nervous system so anyone who often experiences low moods is best served avoiding it. If you drink, drink for the pleasure of it rather than the misconstrued message that alcohol is good for your health.

The link between the consistent overconsumption of alcohol and breast cancer is undeniable. Research has shown this time and time again, and for many years now. Yet we rarely hear about it.

The human body cannot excrete alcohol; it has to be converted into acetaldehyde by the liver, and then the acetaldehyde can be excreted. This is the nasty substance that can give us a headache the day after a big night. If the liver didn't do its job properly and alcohol accumulated in our blood, we can go into a coma and die. Alcohol is that poisonous. And I don't say that lightly. But, thankfully, our liver jumps to action and starts the conversion process and we could carry on. Over time, though, this can take its toll. The trouble is, when we drink daily, or, for some, just regularly, the liver can be so busy dealing with alcohol as its priority, that other substances that the liver has to change so they can be excreted don't get any attention and are recycled. Estrogen and cholesterol are two examples. It is often the reabsorption of these substances that leads to their elevated levels in our bodies—and that can lead to health challenges.

Many people start thinking about their first drink earlier in the day and often when they arrive home they are thirsty and hungry. If you want to cut back or cut out alcohol for a while, or even if you just want to break your habit of regular drinking, have a big glass of water when you first get home and notice if that takes the edge off your desire for alcohol. Most alcoholic drinks contain high levels of sugars, and so have a snack that contains some whole-food fats and see if that alleviates your desire for alcohol.

For other it's the ritual they link to their drinks. When you arrive home, still pour yourself a drink at the time you would normally have a glass of wine, and do what you would normally do. Sit and chat to your partner, make dinner, talk on the phone to a friend. So often we have mentally linked the glass of wine to a pleasurable activity when it is actually the pleasurable activity that we don't want to miss out on! So have sparkling water in a wine glass, with some fresh lime or lemon if that appeals, and add a few more alcohol-free days to your life.

• • • • • • • • • • • • • • • • • • •

Signs your liver needs support

It's time for some liver love! Here's how to recognize signs and symptoms that the liver needs support—and some solutions.

- Liver roll—that increased roll of fat high up under the bra of women, under the pectorals of men

- Tender point in the center of your torso (can indicate gall bladder issues, heartbreak, or massive disappointment); if your gall bladder has been removed, your liver has to make the bile on demand that the gall bladder once stored, so additional liver support is often required

- Very short fuse or temper

- Episodes or feelings of intense anger

- "Liverish," gritty, impatient behavior

- PMS

- Cellulite (also lymphatic)

- Overheating easily

- "Floaters" in your vision (and iron deficiency has been ruled out)

- Waking around 2 a.m.

- Sleep that is worse when you've consumed alcohol the previous evening

- Waking hot in the night

- Not hungry for breakfast when you first get up in the morning

- You prefer to start your day with coffee

- Elevated cholesterol

- Estrogen-dominance symptoms

- You bloat easily

- Drinking alcohol daily

- Daily long-term caffeine consumption

- Elevated blood cholesterol.

LIVER SOLUTIONS

Set yourself a time-based goal when it comes to making these changes. For example, "I will only drink alcohol on weekends for four weeks," or "I will only drink coffee when I go out for breakfast on Sundays."

Take a break from alcohol.

- Only drink on weekends; no alcohol during the week.

- Replace coffee with green or white tea (or, less often, weak, black tea).

- Support the liver with herbs such as:

  > St Mary's Thistle, especially if alcohol is a regular part of your life.

  > Globe artichoke, especially if you have a tendency to constipation, and/or a liver roll, and/or central torso tenderness.

  > Bupleurum, especially if there are clots in the menstrual blood.

  > Schisandra, particularly for its detoxification action (it also supports the adrenals).

- Transform anger into passion by giving a different meaning to a past experience; the energy of anger and passion are similar; they are just directed very differently.

- Drink vegetable juice or a green smoothie most mornings.

- Snack on seeds and nuts.

- Eat less fruit if you eat more than two pieces per day and/or none after morning tea.

- Cut out dairy products for a four-week trial and/or

- Cut out grains (containing gluten) for a four-week trial.

- Take an essential fatty acid supplement: either a good-quality, decent dose of (sustainable, mercury-free) fish oil for reducing cholesterol, or a flax oil, evening primrose oil combination.

- Eat high-zinc foods such as oysters (from clean waters) or take a zinc supplement of zinc picolinate, 15–30mg per day and best taken at night just before bed to maximize absorption.

Remember, it is what you do every day that impacts your health, not what you do sometimes. Just get honest with yourself. And take such good care of yourself that your quality of life is forever excellent. We only have one liver.

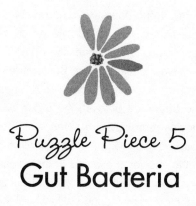

Puzzle Piece 5
Gut Bacteria

This puzzle piece is relatively brief and to the point as far as fat burning is concerned. It is all about the bacterial species that inhabit your large intestine. It is an area in which I have had intense interest since completing my PhD, part of which involved analyzing feces samples from children with autism spectrum disorder (ASD). Not really something to discuss at a dinner party!

What my research—along with countless other scientific studies—taught me was that the way we eat influences the species of gut bacteria that inhabit our colon. Other factors influence this, too. These bacteria eat and produce waste just as a human does. I explored Digestion earlier, but this puzzle piece is all about the colon and the bugs.

The connection between gut bacteria and calories

First, let's explore the influence gut bacteria have on the effect of calories on our body. Wonderful research from 2006[11] demonstrated scientifically what I had observed in my clients and what countless clients already felt to be true—and that is that there seem to be times in our lives when calories behave as if they are worth more in our body. The research took two groups of genetically identical mice with sterile guts; that is, there were no bacteria inhabiting their intestines. The researchers inoculated one group with a range of bacterial species that broadly fit under the name Firmicutes, while the other species were inoculated with Bacteroidetes. Both groups of mice were given an identical number of calories from identical food sources, and (drum roll please!) the group who received the Bacteroidetes species remained the same weight and size while the Firmicutes group gained weight. The mice almost looked "puffy" and "swollen" in the images presented in the scientific paper. This was the first research to show that the types of gut bacteria present in the large bowel may influence the value of calories.

The results of this work went on to be replicated in humans. This study found that people categorized as obese for the purpose of the research had significantly fewer Bacteroidetes in their bowel than lean people in the study. Lean people had a dominance of Bacteroidetes.

Are you one of those people who feel like you only have to look at food for it to end up sticking to you? Do you notice what the people around you eat and wonder how you can be the size you are when you feel as if you eat like a bird? Do you feel the way you eat does not warrant your size? As you have already read in this book, there may be numerous factors at play in this scenario, such as elevated cortisol, estrogen dominance, and/or liver congestion. Science has now shown that the species of bacteria in your large bowel can also play a role.

When I ask people to change their diets for a period of time, usually an initial four weeks, one of the questions in my head is how do I alter this person's gut bacterial profile so their energy improves, their appetite changes (if they overeat in the first place), and their clothes get looser? The first step is to starve the "bad" bugs.

Just like humans, gut bacteria have food preferences, and they have specific "nutritional" requirements. Guess what they thrive on? Sugars! This gives you the biggest reason ever to eliminate refined sugars from your diet for a minimum of four weeks. Not just reduce them. Eliminate them. You must frame it in your head as four tiny weeks out of your very long life. This small chunk of time may provide you with an extraordinarily important answer to your health issues.

If such a challenge feels unattainable, a client who began seeing me when she was 310lbs (140kg)—she volunteered to share her weight—taught me a very effective way to do it. After hearing me speak at a seminar, she identified sugar as her biggest challenge. Cutting sugar back, let alone cutting it out completely, seemed impossible to her and felt like an overwhelming task. She had heard me hark on and on about the enormous importance of greens (especially green leaves), and so instead of starting by cutting sugar out—instead of focusing on eating less of something—she simply focused on eating more: more greens. Within four weeks, she said she no longer even wanted sugar. Her words to me were "it tastes terrible, and I feel like I'm poisoning myself." Extreme perhaps, but you get the message—sugar tastes lousy after you've been eating a lot of green foods for a while, because greens are bitter, and the sugar tastes sickeningly sweet. So up your greens, and watch your desire for sugars fall away. Cutting it out of your diet will change your whole chemistry, as you will see in later chapters.

What many people don't realize is that all carbohydrates are broken down into glucose in the body. Whether those carbohydrates come from sugars or starches, they are all digested and eventually converted into their most basic units: glucose. The body must have a source of glucose, as the brain, kidneys, and red blood cells require glucose for their fuel. My point in ensuring you are clear on this, though, is that today, with the extensive array of processed foods available, it is easy not only to over consume refined sugars but also refined starches; that is, foods made from highly processed, low-nutritional-value grains. To do the work we need to do to address this puzzle piece, refined starches are best omitted for a trial period of four weeks as well. If that feels overwhelming, please don't allow that to stop you taking action. Omitting refined sugars might be your best focus.

Irritable bowel syndrome (IBS)

While I am presenting information about gut bacteria, I want to touch on irritable bowel syndrome (IBS), because a bloated stomach, even though it's different from a fat stomach, can communicate the same message to the brain, particularly to a female one. And studies suggest IBS affects approximately one in five women in many Western countries. I like to say—as with PMS—it is common but it is not normal. It is not how it is supposed to be. Food is not supposed to bloat us.

Regardless of your physical size, if you look down and see a bloated stomach, there is an alarm that screeches inside your head, whether you recognize it or not, "Look how fat you are!" It doesn't matter if you have eaten healthy food that day and exercised, or eaten poorly and done nothing but sit on your bottom, but if you distinctly recall waking that morning with your tummy looking quite OK but now it looks like you've swallowed a football, then it's going to have an effect. Logic disappears at this point. If you were still thinking logically, you would tell yourself that it is not possible to gain a football's worth of fat in a day and that your tummy is simply bloated, to calm down, things will be fine again in the morning, and that it would be good to get to the bottom of your bloatedness. But the potential for that train of thought left the building the moment your brain saw your protruding tummy.

Instead, common reactions in the psyche, especially the female one, might be sudden onset of a really bad mood, overreaction to anything and everything, tears at the drop of a hat, withdrawal, or a major "what the heck" food attack that leaves the pantry bare. Some people are aware of what led to their change in mood. Most are not. And it is worse for those who have been making massive efforts with food and movement. The people who have eaten poorly that day still feel lousy about themselves, but they follow that lousy feeling with thoughts that drive more lousy feelings such as, "Well, what did you expect? You ate cake when you said you weren't going to. You're so hopeless, you have no willpower, and you'll never change." Really non-uplifting sentiments that do not inspire insights that could lead to a change in behavior!

Such reactions raise numerous issues about beliefs and behaviors, many of which are emotional and are explored in Puzzle Piece 9, Emotions. However, on a physical level, which is my focus here, it is essential that we examine why your tummy keeps bloating. Ask yourself:

- Is it related to your menstrual cycle only?

- Does it only happen after you eat lunch? If so, what are you eating for lunch?

- Does your tummy bloat only after an afternoon snack? What are you choosing at this time of day?

- Is it worse when you are stressed? Did it only begin after you went through a great deal of change, positive or not so positive? Did it begin (but perhaps not immediately) after a relationship break-up? Or a period of disordered eating?

- Did it start after an episode of food poisoning or after a holiday where you had a very upset tummy?

My experience with the above scenarios follows.

Menstrual cycle-related bloat

If your tummy only bloats in the lead-up to your period, it is likely to be caused by estrogen dominance. Take the steps outlined on page 96 in Puzzle Piece 3, Sex Hormones.

After-meal bloating

In my experience working with clients, I have learned that there are some foods that are better eaten on an empty stomach if you have challenges with your digestive system. Fruit is one of them. If bloating is an issue for you, only eat fruit first thing in the morning on an empty stomach—none for lunch and none midafternoon. This includes dried fruit. You may find the same thing happens with starchy carbohydrates such as bread. Some people bloat no matter what time of day they eat bread, and, if that is the case, they will usually do well omitting all gluten-containing grains for a four-week period. Others are fine with bread/toast for breakfast but for lunch it is a disaster in their digestive system. Bread is a highly processed food, after all.

All foods containing casein (foods derived from an udder; cow, goat, or sheep, although the latter two tend to be tolerated better than cow's milk) can be significant contributors to a bloated stomach. Remove all sources from your diet for a trial period of four weeks and observe how you feel. If you omit foods for more than four weeks, it is important you consult an experienced health professional to ensure you are not missing out on critical nutrients.

You will like this next bit even less. Coffee can be incredibly bloating for some people. With a milk-based coffee, it may be the cow's milk or, less for some, the soy (soya) milk, but even black coffee will cause some people to bloat. Biochemically, coffee drives both liver and gallbladder action, plus it triggers the adrenals to secrete adrenalin, which can go on to affect another adrenal hormone, called aldosterone, one that determines how much fluid your body retains. Switch to herbal tea or green tea, and give coffee a rest for four weeks. Green tea contains some caffeine (about one-third the caffeine of coffee) but the effects are buffered by another substance in green tea called theanine. Green tea is also packed with antioxidants and has what are believed to be powerful anticancer properties.

Observation is key to this process since your body does not have a voice. Instead it communicates through symptoms and lets you know when it is happy or not. A food that bloats you is, in that moment, not your friend, and your body is simply letting you know. Do not let your head run away with you when you notice this. Remind yourself that just because it bloats you today does not mean you will never eat that food or drink that drink again. It simply means that right now, in this moment, it does not serve you. So take a four-week break from whatever you suspect. No tears, no tantrums, just cut it out for four weeks. You will feel so different when you feed your body precisely what it wants and what nourishes it. Never waste a bloated tummy. Ask it what it wants to tell you, as silly as that may sound. Your body has a wonderful wisdom.

Bloated since a stressful experience

If your tummy changed after a challenging time in your life, it is quite likely that your bloated abdomen was initially due to poor stomach acid production. Now, however, if poor stomach acid production has been ongoing because of an almost low-grade (or high-grade) anxiety inside you, the changes in digestion that were initially caused by poor stomach acid production may have changed the gut bacteria and hence the pH of the large bowel. Follow the solutions given on page 27 in the Digestion chapter, in particular those about stimulating stomach acid and eating in a calm state. Restorative practices will be essential for your gut healing.

Also, return to Puzzle Piece 2, Stress Hormones, again and apply the adrenal support techniques described on page 66. Very importantly, but challenging at times, do your best to eat in a calm state. And you will also often see an improvement in symptoms if you follow the food recommendations from the after-meal bloating section above. If bloating began after heartbreak, ask the discomfort what it wants you to know. You may feel a little odd having a conversation with your tummy, but your body knows the truth, and you might be surprised at the message it has for you.

Bloated since food poisoning episode or upset tummy while traveling

Despite negative stool tests, I have seen this health picture frequently. Where once they had an iron gut, this person now feels like they react to everything. Even if you had forgotten that a gastroenteritis episode began your digestive system challenges, I suggest you:

- Discuss having a *Helicobacter pylori* test with your general practitioner (GP/MD).

- Take a herbal anti-parasitic tablet or liquid, even if your stool test came back negative. Be guided by a health professional, but you usually need relatively high doses three times a day, and you need to take them for a two-month period. If a parasite infection is the basis of your ongoing tummy trouble, the natural medicine must be taken for the full two months, as initially only the live parasites are killed by the herbs. As unpleasant as this is to think about, the parasites will have laid eggs in your bowel, and you want the herbs in your gut at the ready, in order to get rid of them immediately as they hatch, if this is the case.

- Dietary change as outlined above can be very useful in this situation until the gut has healed. What has become known as a "caveman"-style diet (or the Paleolithic or Primal diet; please note, there is no one way people from the Paleolithic era ate; in a modern dietary sense, this name refers to a way of eating primarily whole foods), that is both milk- and grain-free can be beneficial. This way of eating also includes broths, which are highly nourishing for the gut. The Specific Carbohydrate Diet (SCD) has also been noted to have excellent results for gut health challenges and to alter gut bacteria profiles.

- A low-FODMAPs diet has also been shown to be highly beneficial for people with gut-based health challenges. (FODMAPs is an acronym referring to Fermentable,

Oligosaccharides, Disaccharides, Monosaccharides and Polyols.) These are complex names for a collection of molecules found in food that can be poorly absorbed by some people. When the molecules are poorly absorbed in the small intestine of the digestive tract, these molecules then continue their journey along the digestive tract, arriving at the large intestine, where they act as a food source to the bacteria that live there. The bacteria then digest/ferment these FODMAPs and can cause symptoms of IBS. The fermentation action of gut bacteria on FODMAPs can also be one reason why some people feel better without fruit (or with only small amounts of specific fruits) when they have gut or autoimmune symptoms.

The no-good bug... streptococcus

There is a bacterial species that I must mention, and I dislike it intensely. It is called *streptococcus*, and my experience in the lab, as well as working with people and their health, has taught me that no good comes from this bug.

It is the bug that causes tonsillitis and ear infections. It is often the basis of pneumonia and other respiratory infections. It lives in our sinuses and builds houses around itself so we can't evacuate it easily. It produces many toxins, as well as lactic acid—more acid to add to our already acidic lifestyles and loads. When our heads are full of mucus, especially when we are young, it can be difficult to cough up all of the sputum, and so we cannot help but swallow some. Our stomach acid is supposed to be super-acidic enough to sterilize anything bacterial that we swallow, yet, as outlined on page 6 in the chapter on digestion, the pH of the stomach is often too high to perform adequate sterilization. So the strep is able to move through the stomach and take up residence wherever it likes. And there it lives, often forever, in our colon.

Learn to know your gut bugs

As well as being able to categorize gut bacteria into the groups Firmicutes and Bacteroidetes, we can classify them into those that love oxygen, known as "aerobes," and those that don't use oxygen, called "anaerobes." For good health, of the aerobic flora in our large bowel, 70 to 90 percent need to be E. coli. It is believed that "reasonable" health can be maintained as long as there is 5 percent or less of the streptococcus species. I have analyzed stool samples from countless people from many walks of life, with an array of health challenges as well as good health—adults and children—and I have seen aerobic flora counts of streptococcus at 100 percent of the aerobic flora with zero E. coli. Or, less extremely, I have seen strep counts of 70 percent and E. coli of 30 percent.

Mostly due to my work with children with autism, I have seen firsthand that strep is nasty. ASD behaviors decrease significantly with less strep in the gut. In adults, strep makes them wet and mucusy mouth-breathers, which negatively affects their blood chemistry (predominantly bicarbonate and the anion gap).

Of the bacterial genres of Firmicutes and Bacteroidetes (remembering that Firmicutes are linked to fat storage and Bacteroidetes to leanness), strep falls into the Firmicute division. So after all of these years of treating strep in the gut of my clients, knowing they would feel better, breathe better, and that their clothes would get looser, what researching this book has shown me is that all along I have been significantly reducing the Firmicute load in the gut of my clients with the dietary changes I suggest. Isn't the body amazing?

Signs your gut bacteria needs to be addressed

- You have taken antibiotics and no probiotics

- You feel like you eat like a bird and gain weight, while others seem to eat far more than you and not gain weight

- You identified with numerous signs that your digestive system needs support *(see page 25)*, including bloating/gut distention, excessive or odorous flatulence, recurring bad breath, gut pain, or gut gurgling sounds

- You have had food poisoning and never felt the same since

- You traveled and experienced an upset tummy (gastrointestinal infection), and haven't felt well since

- Your mood changes inexplicably

- You have IBS

- You feel like you are becoming more and more sensitive to foods

- You had recurring streptococcus infections as a child

- You have strong Irish heritage and you eat gluten-containing grains

- You have an autoimmune disease or a family member/s does/do.

GUT BACTERIA SOLUTIONS

Apply any or all of the solutions offered in this chapter, including herbal parasite treatments, refined sugar-free diet trial, dairy-free diet trial, gluten-free diet trial, grain-free diet trial, or *Helicobacter pylori* tests. An experienced health professional is best to guide you with this. In addition, you may find the following solutions helpful.

- A caveman-style diet can be highly appropriate to help change the gut bacterial ratios: plenty of vegetables, particularly greens, small servings of red meat, chicken, fish (if you eat them), eggs, nuts, seeds and nourishing whole-food fats. The Specific Carbohydrate

Diet or FODMAPs can also be very helpful. Use these diets as a trial, not necessarily forever. If you restrict your diet for more than four weeks, you will need to see an experienced health professional to ensure you are meeting your nutritional needs.

- You may "know" that grains are not your friends. If so, cut them out for four weeks to see how you feel.

- Use 100 percent aloe vera juice to start your day as this can help put the very important mucus lining back on the wall of the bowel. Bone broths are also highly nourishing and can add additional gut healing support.

- Useful antimicrobial/immune system herbs include:

  > Golden seal

  > Echinacea

  > Barberry

  > Astragalus

  > Olive leaf

  > Chinese wormwood

  > Black walnut

  > Andrographis

- To use these herbs, it is essential that you seek individual advice from a qualified medical herbalist.

- It is also essential that you use your bowels daily before using antimicrobial herbs, as you want to eliminate the waste easily.

- Explore the use of colon hydrotherapy from an experienced practitioner.

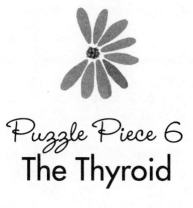

Puzzle Piece 6
The Thyroid

The thyroid gland is a little butterfly-shaped gland that sits in your throat area. It makes hormones that play an enormous role in your metabolic rate as well as temperature regulation. Every day of my working life I meet people who exhibit virtually every symptom of an underactive thyroid, yet their blood test results demonstrate that everything is in the "normal" range. More on "normal" ranges later.

The production of thyroid hormones involves a cascade of signals, and glands other than the thyroid are also involved. This means that if you have a problem with thyroid hormone levels or with debilitating symptoms indicating something is awry with your thyroid function then it is essential to get to the heart of the matter so treatment can be appropriately targeted.

The thyroid hormone cascade

The thyroid function cascade begins with the hypothalamus, a gland that makes a hormone that sends a signal to the pituitary gland, the tiny gland that sits at the base of your brain, which we've already seen produces hormones involved in menstruation. The pituitary in turn makes a hormone called thyroid stimulating hormone (TSH) that signals the thyroid to make one if its hormones, known simply as T4 (thyroxine).

T4 is found in the blood in two forms, namely T4 and free T4 (FT4). They are the same hormone, except one is "free" to enter tissues and the other is bound up and unable to enter tissues, which is where the work needs to be done. However, T4 and FT4 are inactive hormones, and must be converted into the active thyroid hormone called T3 (triiodothyronine). It is T3 that drives your metabolic rate and capacity to burn body fat. The flow chart below illustrates the hormonal cascade.

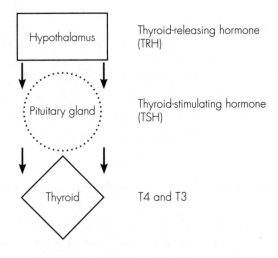

Figure 13: The thyroid hormone cascade
Signaling begins with the hypothalamus followed by the pituitary,
which then in turn signals the thyroid gland to make its hormones.

There are a number of nutrients essential in the production of optimal levels of thyroid hormones. Iodine and selenium are both vital minerals to this process of conversion that literally lights up your metabolic rate. Many people today get very little iodine and selenium in their diets as the majority of soils in the Western world do not contain these trace minerals.

Iron is also critical to good thyroid function and iron deficiency remains as the most common nutrient deficiency among women of menstruation age. This is unacceptable to me, as we know how to resolve this and the consequences of low iron levels are extensive. In a state of iron deficiency, instead of efficiently converting the inactive T4 into the active T3 hormone, too much T4 is converted into a different hormone known as reverse T3 (rT3), which does not have the same metabolism-driving effects as T3. So when you think about specific nutrients for good thyroid function, think iodine, selenium, and iron. I spend significant time exploring optimal thyroid function at my women's health weekends as it is such a challenge for more and more women these days and seeing the moments of realization flash across their faces, as they understand what may have been occurring for them, is a gift to witness.

The thyroid gland can become overactive, known as hyperthyroidism, or underactive, known as hypothyroidism, and it is the latter scenario that can lead to weight gain that is incredibly difficult to shift until this issue is addressed. Some people's blood results suggest that they swing between an underactive and an overactive situation.

The thyroid gland is also susceptible to autoimmune diseases, meaning your immune system, which is supposed to defend you from infection, starts to see the thyroid gland as a foreign particle, like a germ, and attacks it, leading to a change in its function. This can lead to either the overactive picture (with autoimmune involvement this is known as Graves' disease) or an underactive picture (known as Hashimoto's thyroiditis with autoimmune involvement). Infection, poor liver function, iodine, selenium, and iron deficiencies, as well as estrogen dominance or elevated cortisol, are all major factors that can initiate this process. Reread that list and think about what you have already learned from earlier chapters. It is important to work out the path that leads someone to altered thyroid function, for behind the "why" lies most of the answer and hence the pathway out of the dysfunction.

Which factors stand out for you? Sometimes all of the above apply. Never fear, there are solutions.

Hypothyroidism: Underactive thyroid gland function

Because this book is about explaining what has to come together for us to be able to burn body fat, I will stay focused on hypothyroidism (underactive thyroid) and what can lead to it. As far as an overactive thyroid goes, I will simply leave it at this: in my experience, stress, specifically the pace of life and what people demand of their body, is the major factor in the development of hyperthyroidism. The people I've worked with who have successfully returned their thyroid function to normal (from being overactive), and had a complete remission of their symptoms, have literally changed their life. They usually change their jobs and, if that is not possible, they completely change their approach and attitude to life. It has been inspiring to witness in my clients. Louise Hay suggests in *You Can Heal Your Life* there is a feeling of "rage at being left out," and encourages people to affirm "I am the center of my life, and I approve of myself and all that I see."

Back to hypothyroidism and its typical symptoms, which include:

- Gradual weight increase over months for no apparent reason

- Often feeling cold, sometimes cold in your bones and as if you can't get warm

- Tendency to constipation

- Tendency to depressed mood, forgetfulness, and a sense of being easily confused

- Hair loss or hair drier than previously

- Menstrual problems

- Difficulty conceiving

- Beyond tired, you are fatigued

- Headaches

Let's explore the roads to an underactive thyroid and where to begin to support your thyroid health.

Infection and poor liver detoxification

A history of glandular fever (Epstein-Barr virus, also known as mononucleosis), for example, is a common road to hypothyroidism, as is liver congestion (described on page 116 in Puzzle Piece 4, The Liver). Treatment of both of these roads involves taking excellent care of the liver. Apply the liver-loving strategies outlined in the liver chapter. Additionally, astragalus is an excellent herb to use for a chronic infection background if a herbalist agrees this will meet your needs.

Mineral deficiencies

Since hypothyroidism can be influenced by deficiencies in selenium, iodine, and iron, choose foods that are rich in these minerals. Eat Brazil nuts daily for selenium. Use good-quality salt, ensuring it contains iodine (check the label) and/or cook with seaweeds such as Kombu for iodine. Food sources of iron include beef, lamb, eggs, mussels, sardines, lentils, green leafy vegetables, and dates. There is a small amount of iron in many foods, so eating a varied diet is important. And remember that absorption is enhanced by vitamin C. If you do not eat animal foods, do not assume you are iron deficient. For some vegetarians, their body utilizes the iron from vegetables sources very efficiently. It is worth having your iron levels tested next time you see your GP/MD.

The other option is to take a supplement that covers these nutrients. There are some excellent thyroid support capsules on the market so seek out one of these if it appeals. Regarding iron, it can be good to have a test before you supplement, as overloading on iron is not good. But if you are deficient it can be challenging and a very slow process to get your iron levels up without supplementation. So it is good to know your blood levels of this mineral. Many iron supplements are constipating, but most people find this doesn't happen with liquid iron supplements.

Here's some more on iodine from a magazine article I wrote... just so you know how important this is!

Iodine

Iodine is a trace mineral so essential to our health that our body begins to shut down without it. Our thyroid gland loves iodine, and it cannot make thyroid hormones without it. Symptoms of an underactive thyroid include a deep tiredness and sluggish, heavy feeling; dry skin or hair; feelings of cold; a tendency to be constipated; puffy eyes; and a tendency to a depressed mood. Increasing dietary iodine intake can make a difference, if poor thyroid function is the result of iodine deficiency.

Thyroid hormones essentially determine our metabolic rate as adults and our growth as children. Iodine is also essential to the IQ of the developing brain in utero and, sadly, studies are now showing that some children in the Western world are suffering from such low iodine levels that their IQ is being detrimentally affected.

Why is this so?

Soil is a poor source of iodine, and if a nutrient is not in the soil it cannot be in our food. New Zealand, for example, has volcanic soil, which has never contained any iodine. While the soil may not be a good source of iodine, the sea is somewhat better.

Food sources of iodine include all of the seaweeds, which you can add to soups, stews, casseroles, and salads to give them a subtle salty flavor while imparting all of the nutritional value of the minerals. A form of seaweed commonly eaten is nori, used frequently in sushi. Iodine is in small amounts in seafood, but even eating seafood every day will not provide you with adequate amounts of iodine. Plus, sadly, these days, we have to consider the heavy metal content of seafood and eating it daily is not recommended. We must therefore be conscious of how we obtain our iodine.

Salt was first iodized in 1924; however, it tended to go out of "fashion" with the advent of rock salts and Celtic sea salt. Although Celtic sea salt offers the additional benefits of a broad range of trace minerals, many brands lack iodine. You need to check the label of the salt you use. The concern with conventional iodized salts, however, is that most brands contain anti-caking agents that tend to have other additives that may not be ideal for human health.

The impact of iodine therapy for the maintenance of healthy breast tissue has been widely reported, although it is rarely discussed. The ovaries concentrate iodine, and studies have shown that the ovaries in an iodine-deficient state produce a form of estrogen associated with breast cancer. This has been shown to be reversible once iodine levels are optimal again.

Iodine is a difficult mineral to test for. Accurate tests require you to collect 24 hours' worth of urine, and, remarkably, not all countries offer this testing.

Adults require 150mcg of iodine per day to prevent deficiency. It is far more beneficial, however, to individualize doses. Often higher amounts are initially needed to treat a deficient state, and this can be easily done with one to three drops of a good-quality liquid iodine solution per *day, available from some health food shops or through a compounding pharmacist. It is best to obtain specific advice from a qualified health professional to learn how best to meet your individual needs, as you can overdose on iodine.*

● ● ● ● ● ● ● ● ● ● ● ● ● ● ● ● ● ● ●

Estrogen dominance

Too much estrogen suppresses thyroid function while optimal progesterone levels support its function. Apply the strategies for dealing with estrogen dominance if you suspect that this is the basis for your challenge with your thyroid gland. It is also important to note that knowing what led to an underactive thyroid gland is critical to your healing. For example, if long-term estrogen dominance has suppressed your thyroid function, no amount of iodine will resolve it. Restoring iodine status will support a thyroid gland that has become underactive through poor dietary iodine intake, though.

Elevated cortisol brought on by stress

Elevated cortisol as a result of stress decreases the levels of the active, fat-burning thyroid hormone T3, which then slows your metabolism. Added to this, high levels of cortisol urge your body to break down muscle to provide glucose for your brain, and reducing your muscle mass slows your metabolic rate as well. In the absence of stress, a healthy body converts FT4 into T3, but with elevated cortisol levels, the conversion of FT4 to T3 decreases.

Poor conversion of FT4 to active T3 also occurs if you restrict your food intake. Your body assumes that you must be starving, and therefore it must slow down the metabolic rate to preserve those precious fat stores. It may be frustrating, but your body's primary goal is always for survival.

Elevated cortisol also inhibits the release of TSH from the pituitary—with less TSH the body produces less FT4. Apply the strategies for high cortisol outlined on pages 48–49 in Puzzle Piece 2, Stress Hormones, if this scenario rings true for you. Poor thyroid function can also lead to elevated cholesterol, and, if this is the case, once thyroid function has been treated, the cholesterol returns to normal.

Thyroid medications

Typically today, if someone has been diagnosed with an underactive thyroid, they are prescribed thyroxine (T4). Some people feel brilliant on this medication and all of their hypothyroid symptoms disappear, including their weight gain. If this has not happened for you despite taking this medication, you may want to consider a different approach. After years of taking thyroxine, it will not suddenly start to work if it hasn't yet.

There are numerous brands of thyroxine on the market. If you want to stick with conventional medicine, tell your general practitioner you feel lousy on your current medication and that you would like to try a different drug. I have hundreds of clients who were happily taking one form of thyroxine and when the thyroid medication that is subsidized was changed to a different brand, many of their symptoms returned. Explore this even if your blood levels of TSH, FT4, and T3 are "normal," but you still have symptoms.

In my opinion, an excellent option when it comes to hypothyroidism is whole thyroid extract (WTE). This is taken instead of any synthetic medication and, unlike the synthetics providing only one of the thyroid hormones, WTE provides all of the thyroid hormones. It is essential that you see your doctor about this and, if you so choose, be guided in the transition from a synthetic to the WTE, which is made by a compounding pharmacist. Like all medicines, WTE doesn't suit everyone, so be guided by your body and an experienced health professional with this.

If you have not been diagnosed with a thyroid illness, but you exhibit numerous symptoms, do not rely solely on your blood test results to determine if your thyroid is underactive. Work with a health professional who will treat the symptoms, not the blood, and who will monitor both your symptoms and the blood work as you explore treatments. I learned this in a powerful way with a client whose story melts my heart.

Case Study

The importance of testing thyroid antibodies is best demonstrated with this story. A precious lady arrived at my practice for assistance with her health, and when I asked how I could help, she burst into tears and said she had known she had an underactive thyroid for about 30 years. Patricia's blood tests always came back as normal, and no one would treat her. She had gained over 220lbs over 30 years, and it all began when her mother passed away. Patricia said she had eaten poorly for about three to four months after her death, and put on weight, but her grief gradually eased and, as it did, she started to eat better again, as she always had. But nothing changed. Her size kept increasing. So then she didn't just eat well, she signed up for a gym membership, and she started to eat even better. When I saw her, Patricia was unable to exercise due to knee pain from carrying so much weight (her description, and she thought she was "about 400lbs"), but she still ate in a way that did not warrant her size.

Of course Patricia had a huge amount of unresolved grief and of course there had been times when she hadn't eaten very well. She had, at times, become incredibly frustrated that despite her efforts nothing would shift. But she had also had plenty of months and years of making extraordinary efforts for no reward.

Given that Patricia ticked every box when it came to symptoms of an underactive thyroid, I decided to request fresh blood tests and include thyroid antibodies, specifically anti-thyroid peroxidase and anti-thyroglobulin. Having been taught throughout my education that it was highly unlikely for thyroid antibodies to be elevated and an issue if thyroid hormone levels were in the normal range, I could understand why Patricia's thyroid antibodies had not been tested—but from a symptoms perspective I could not.

To cut a very long story short, despite her latest thyroid hormone levels being in the "normal" range, albeit skewed one way (discussed below), Patricia's antibodies were the highest I have ever seen. To put this in context, the "normal" range for both antibodies in this national laboratory is less than 50 (<50). Patricia's thyroid peroxidase and thyroglobulin were both greater than 6,500 (>6,500)—off the scale and through the roof. When I phoned her to tell her, she was at first thrilled that all along there had been a reason for how lousy she had felt. She told me later that anger then surfaced for a life she felt she'd missed out on because it was not picked up. She had remained very shy, which she blamed on her size, and on reflection was very sad that she had not met a partner with whom to share her life.

She decided to seek out the most natural approach she could for her very underactive thyroid, and after considerable weight fell off her over the first three months, she booked her first overseas vacation. There is always a why. You just have to find it.

• • • • • • • • • • • • • • • • • •

Blood tests and "normal" ranges

The concept of a normal range is necessary, as cutoff points help indicate when something may be abnormal. Plus normal ranges guide us. I have great concerns, however, when we base the entire future of a person's health on blood tests alone. The symptoms the body presents are a guide, just as normal ranges are a guide, and a thorough health professional will bring all of this information together to gain a broader picture to help determine what might be going on for a person.

According to Dr. Karen Coates, an insightful and pioneering general practitioner and co-author of *Embracing The Warrior: An Essential Guide for Women*, the normal range for some blood tests is calculated periodically by each pathology laboratory to ensure that the reference range printed on the test results is "accurate." On the morning of this day, the first 100 blood samples received are tested for their (in this case) TSH levels in order to determine the reference range. Or it might be iron levels, for example. But! Why do people usually have blood tests? Is it because they are feeling particularly sprightly that day? No! Most often, the precise opposite is true! Yet it seems we base our "normal" ranges on these figures.

Furthermore, it is also important to understand how the "average" amount of a particular nutrient or hormone is calculated. Mathematically, the top reference point is calculated to be "two standard deviations" above the average, while the bottom figure is "two standard deviations" below the average. The arbitrary rules of this method dictate that 95 percent of the 100 blood samples taken must fall into the "normal" range. The statistical definition of standard deviations insists that only four or five results may fall outside this reference range, two samples below and two above.

The two points I want to make are: first, the reference ranges for some blood parameters are getting broader. The normal range for TSH (in my country) when I wrote the first draft of this book was 0.4 to 4.0. The normal range has since been expanded to 0.3 to 5.0 only four months after. As mentioned later, people at either end of this blood range will typically look and feel completely different and they will more than likely exhibit thyroid symptoms. If they are symptom-free, no problem, but my concern is that if we base treatment on the blood work alone and leave people to live with their symptoms with their result skewed to one end of the normal range, we are risking, not optimizing, their health. This brings me to my next point, which is that you can see from the start that this process is flawed, given it is done on individuals who are unwell. It is more challenging to create optimal health, prevent disease, and maximize quality of life for people when they are being guided with their blood tests to fall into a potentially unhealthy normal range.

Your blood tests

I urge you to get copies of your own blood tests and look for results being skewed to one end of the normal range. Let me explain.

The normal range for TSH where I live is 0.3 to 5.0. Although those numbers may seem small, someone with a TSH of 0.3 tends to feel and look completely different from someone with a TSH of 5.0. Additionally, if your results are not actually outside the normal range, you will usually be told (well-meaningly) that there is no problem with your thyroid. A common picture I see is a TSH of 2.5 or greater screaming out to the thyroid gland to make FT4. FT4 normal levels are (where I live) 10 to 20 units and usually, for someone with symptoms of hypothyroidism, their FT4 will be 11. This person typically feels exhausted, has trouble naturally using their bowels daily, has dry skin, very low motivation, brain fog, and their clothes are gradually getting tighter. Their thyroid needs support.

In this case, and depending on their dietary intake, I tend to start with iodine and selenium and sometimes iron, along with adrenal support, a grain-free diet, and a big chat about their beliefs and what their perception is of what life is like for them. Louise Hay teaches that thyroid problems represent feelings and beliefs around humiliation and feeling like you never get to do what you want to do (how many mothers does that describe?). Louise suggests someone with thyroid problems subconsciously asks, "When is it going to be my turn?" She suggests you develop a new thought pattern of "I move beyond old limitations and now allow myself to express freely and creatively." Underneath diagnosed hypothyroidism, Louise suggests, are feelings of hopelessness, a feeling of being stifled, and a sense of giving up. She suggests you develop a new thought pattern of "I create a new life with new rules that totally support me."

I include this information to offer you a whole picture of your thyroid health, from the conventional function of hormones and glands and blood tests; through the nutritional supports that are essential, including iodine and selenium; to the metaphysical. Somewhere among these three approaches lies your answer, not necessarily in one or the other. I urge you to explore all three.

Signs your thyroid needs support

Please note that many of the symptoms of an overactive thyroid are often the opposite of an underactive thyroid; some people may experience both conditions in their lifetime. Given an underactive thyroid is more related to being overweight than an overactive thyroid, this piece of the puzzle focuses predominantly on the underactive state.

Signs of an underactive thyroid

- "Unexplained" weight gain

- Feeling cold in your bones, or you notice you are colder than others around you—you are the first to put on a jumper

- When you read symptoms of an underactive thyroid they resonate with you, yet you are told your blood test results are fine; when you see them though, they tend to be skewed to one end of the "normal" range

- You have a tendency toward constipation, dry skin, and brittle hair

- You have long-term estrogen dominance symptoms, such as PMS

- You feel weary to your bones; you are beyond tired. Your body feels heavy and lethargic

- Your reactions to stimuli—both physical and emotional—feel slow

- You crave salt

- You crave coffee and it doesn't amp you up—your brain feels slightly more functional after you have it

- Your groin aches

- Your voice has changed; it is husky on occasions, particularly when you are extra tired (can also be a sign that the adrenals need support)

- You feel like you retain fluid

- Tendency toward a depressed mood, forgetfulness, and a sense of being easily confused

- Hair loss

- Difficulty conceiving

- Challenges with menstruation

- Recurrent headaches

- You've had your gallbladder removed

- Chronic stress

- Family history of thyroid dysfunction or disease

- Family history of autoimmune conditions

- You have been diagnosed with adrenal fatigue or another condition involving the endocrine system; or you have been previously diagnosed with an autoimmune condition

- You wonder when it will be your turn—when you will be able to do what you want to do, rather than what others want or need from you.

Signs of an overactive thyroid

- "Unexplained" weight loss

- Overheating easily

- You have a tendency to "unexplained" loose stools

- Rapid heartbeat or heart palpitations

- You are amped-up regularly and tend toward anxious feelings

- Your eyes are bulging forward from the eye sockets

- Chronic stress

- Family history of thyroid dysfunction or disease

- Family history of autoimmune conditions

- You have been diagnosed with adrenal fatigue or another condition involving the endocrine system; or you have been previously diagnosed with an autoimmune condition.

THYROID SOLUTIONS

Solutions are scattered throughout this chapter, so please go back and reread it a second time to create your plan of action to optimize thyroid function. My additional suggestions are, as follows:

- Go on a grain-free diet trial for a minimum of four weeks. Gut health often needs to be at the heart of thyroid treatments, particularly if there are antibodies present in the blood.

- If you *love* dairy products and the idea of going without cheese makes you wonder if you could, then do it! It is often what we love (not just like) to eat that can be a problem. Do a four-week dairy-free trial if this is the case.

- Have an experienced health professional assess your diet for iodine and selenium intake, and have a blood test to examine not only thyroid parameters, but also iron status.

- Support liver and gallbladder function to assist with bowel elimination. Globe artichoke is particularly good for "thyroid" people.

- Refer to the advice about estrogen dominance.

- Adrenal support is almost always essential, especially when beginning to treat the thyroid. Refer to page 65 in Puzzle Piece 2, Stress Hormones, to refresh on adrenal support strategies.

- You will probably crave coffee. Please explore taking a four-week break and observe how you feel at the end of this period. Use green tea, which has a low caffeine level, herbal tea, or dandelion tea instead.

- If you have a diagnosed thyroid condition and you are on synthetic medication but your symptoms are still present, explore transitioning to whole thyroid extract under medical supervision.

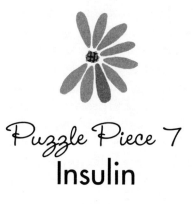

Puzzle Piece 7
Insulin

The pancreas is another gland (technically it is a "gland organ") that makes a hormone intricately linked to body-fat burning or accumulation. Insulin is made by the pancreas, and it is a type of growth hormone, hence its capacity to drive fat storage. We make insulin when we eat. Carbohydrates elicit the largest production while protein drives only a small amount of insulin release, which is usually offset by another hormone that protein elicits called glucagon, which acts in the opposite way to insulin. Consuming dietary fats does not drive an insulin response.

People have become confused about and fearful of carbs, yet it's imperative that we consume some carbohydrates since they are vital to the function of our brain, kidneys, and red blood cells. So how do we optimize carbohydrate intake while still burning fat?

How carbs can make you fat—or not

When you consume carbohydrates, whether they are starchy or sweet carbs, they are broken down into glucose. Sources of carbohydrates include bread, pasta, rice, all types of potatoes, and the other starchy vegetables (including pumpkin and corn), fruit, dairy products, candy (sweets and chocolate), cakes, biscuits (cookies), pastries, honey, maple syrup, and sugar. I have found it fascinating to ask audiences to shout out sources of carbohydrates over the years. Today, the only carbs audiences tend to identify are the starches (bread and potato are the first two words out of their mouths virtually every time), which I believe is the result of the high-protein diet era. When I asked audiences to name sources of carbs 17 years ago, the first and almost only word out of their mouths was sugar. Back then, fat was still the "enemy" of the public health nutrition messages, and the public believed that as long as there was very little fat in a food, then it had to be good.

Bread and pasta are high in what were known as complex carbohydrates and very low in fat, and people ate them by the bucketload. Back then there was still some wariness about sugar, as it had been hailed as the only enemy in the late 1970s on the back end of the previous high-protein diet age. You see, nutrition information moves in cycles, and it will continue to do so. To avoid getting caught in the latest fad, I remind you that nature gets it right, and it is human intervention that gets it wrong and makes food less nourishing and sustaining. My point here is that starch-based foods are carbs but so is anything that tastes sweet, unless it has been flavored by artificial sweeteners (*see also page 167 for more on this topic*) or stevia, a beautifully sweet herb.

Glucose from the carbohydrates ends up in your bloodstream after digestion, and your body identifies that blood sugar levels have been elevated. Your body does not like it when blood glucose goes high, as too much sugar in the blood can damage the lining of the blood vessels, in a similar way to a free radical (*described on page 111, in Puzzle Piece 4, The Liver*). To protect the blood vessels from damage, the pancreas secretes insulin into the blood. It is the job of insulin to remove the excess glucose from the blood so that homeostasis (balance) returns to the blood. The health and contents of the blood must be maintained at all costs.

Insulin first takes the glucose to the muscles and the liver, where it is stored as glycogen, places from which it can be released easily when we need a fast source of energy if we haven't eaten for a while. But the size of our muscles is finite, meaning they have their storage limit. Once they are full of glycogen, if more sugar from the blood needs to be removed, insulin will transport it to guess where? The fat cells. Fat cells have an infinite capacity to expand.

An essential point to make here is that our muscle mass is critical. Do not allow yourself to lose muscle from this point forward in your life. At best, increase your muscle mass. At least, maintain it where it is today. Given the glycogen storage capacity of muscles and the ready source of energy they offer, coupled with the metabolism-driving power of muscles, I cannot encourage you enough to grow them. You do not need to become a body builder. You do not need to lift huge amounts of weight. I suggest you focus on strengthening the muscles housed in your core. Of course you can also work on the pretty ones that everyone can see, but make sure your core gets attention. Think about this. All of your organs that keep you alive, other than your brain, are housed inside your torso. These organs are held in place by muscles. Over time, due to gravity, poor posture and poor lifestyle choices, these muscles want to go south and, when this happens, they no longer work as efficiently as they once did. Pilates, yoga, and qi gong are all excellent for core strength, and you can even activate your core while walking sometimes for a little extra bonus. Bring awareness to how you hold yourself and how you move.

Food and insulin

Exploring the human history of food helps guide us with what to eat, especially when it comes to managing insulin levels. The only carbohydrates humans once ate were legumes, pulses (e.g., lentils), and berries, and later root vegetables. These days, there are over 3,000 snack food items alone on the average grocery store's shelves, and this number is growing constantly. None of these packaged foods are what I call "low human intervention" (low HI) foods. Even white bread looks nothing like the stalk of wheat from which it came. If you showed a four-year-old child a stalk of wheat and a piece of white bread, do you think that four-year-old could tell you that the stalk of wheat made the white bread? Unlikely, as they are not even the same color. That stalk of wheat has been bleached, rolled, and pummeled to create that piece of white bread, so much so that all of the nutrition that was present in the original stalk of wheat has been removed and, for that slice of white bread to have any goodness at all, the nutrients have to be added back synthetically. And just as an aside, how did you make glue when you were at school? With flour and water. Now, they package it up and sell it to us.

I am not saying don't ever eat white bread. If you love it, buy it fresh from a good-quality baker, who uses no preservatives, perhaps on a Saturday morning, or better still, buy it fortnightly or even better still, monthly, and enjoy it. Remember, it is what you do every day that has the greatest impact on your health, not what you do sometimes. If you love it, eat it. Just not bucketloads and not every day. And if you need to have a four-week break from grains because of an inkling you might have got from information earlier in this book, then take your break and bring it back on occasions if you want to. You may feel so good without it though, that you never want to go back. It's your call.

It is big surges of insulin on and off over the day or constantly high circulating insulin that cause the problem when it comes to fat burning. If you have spent months committed to exercising and eating well with little or no reward, have your blood glucose level as well as your blood insulin level tested. I have had clients with perfect blood glucose levels but their bodies are making huge amounts of insulin to keep their blood glucose inside the normal range, and you never know this until you test the insulin. No matter how much you exercise or how seemingly amazingly you eat, you will not access your fat stores to burn in this biochemical state. Insulin must be addressed.

Rushing woman's syndrome

A typical pattern of food intake that I witness regularly is this: You get up in the morning, inhale some sort of processed breakfast cereal, and race out the door to work. Your blood sugar soars, and your pancreas subsequently releases a surge of insulin. *Welcome to fat storage situation number one of your day.*

You take shallow breaths all morning due to the perceived pressures in your day. After your peak in blood sugar from your hurried processed-food breakfast, by mid-morning your blood sugar plummets, and concentration levels are waning. You are relieved when you look at your watch and see it is 10:30 a.m. You haven't achieved very much in your day until now other than trying to get on top of emails that you actually never seem to get on top of, but at least it is time for a break, an opportunity to get away from your desk, either with colleagues or by yourself, and head to the nearest coffee cart or café. You justify your desire, and subsequent purchase of a muffin, along with your large double shot skinny milk latte, by telling yourself that you have a big day ahead and you'll probably go to the gym later anyway. *Welcome to fat storage situation number 2 of your day.*

You return to your desk and push on with some work, but, after a couple of hours, you are fidgety again and want lunch. Your blood sugar has come down from the high brought on by your mid-morning snack. You look at your watch again... thank goodness! It's lunchtime! And out you go for lunch. You know you feel better in your tummy on days when you don't eat bread for lunch, but you tell yourself that you are busy and you need to be quick. A sandwich, bagel, or a roll is always quick and easy. You inhale it. Then you want something sweet. *Hmmm. Chocolate? No, not yet. Dried fruit for now*. And, on the inside, your blood sugar and consequently your insulin level surge again. *Welcome to fat storage situation number 3.*

Within half an hour, you feel utterly exhausted, probably bloated, and you are berating yourself because you feel fat. You are, in fact, simply bloated but your discomfort and the wind building in your tummy, coupled with your swollen abdomen, makes you feel gross. You work in an open-plan office, so you are conscious of hanging onto that wind in case it has an odor (men don't seem to worry about this in the way women do!). And so even though your colleagues may be (unknowingly) grateful, the bloating and hence the size of your tummy increases over the afternoon.

Headspace and hormones

The psychological process that goes on in your head, particularly if you are a woman, after lunch when you reflect on what you have consumed that morning, is incredibly detrimental to your health and your cortisol levels and, hence, your waistline. You feel like all you did was eat all morning and sit on your bottom. You think about the dress you were planning to fit into to wear to an event three weeks from now. Even though all you have done is eat breakfast, a muffin, a coffee, and a roll, in that moment, you believe that you will never fit into that dress and even though you thought you would go to the gym that evening, having not achieved very much over your morning, you know you will work late and not go. You think about the gym membership that cost you half a month's pay and that you haven't used it for the last three months, and you feel useless. You think again about the "massive" (as perceived by you) amounts of food you have eaten so far that day, and you berate yourself and your swollen abdomen. Then! Lightbulb! A thought that suddenly makes you feel better flashes into your mind. You suddenly feel back in control. What was that thought? "I won't eat a snack this afternoon!"

You feel better, because you have found a way out of your perceived eating frenzy and expanding (bloated) waistline. But your blood sugar and insulin picture over your morning resembled a rollercoaster, so how do you expect your blood sugar picture to be any different than it was in the morning? The answer is it won't be. By 3 or 4 p.m., your blood sugar has plummeted again, and you feel exhausted. The momentary elation from your "no afternoon snack" thought has vaporized and you are now "starving," to the point that you could eat your arm off. Your blood *sugar* is rock bottom. So, instinctively, what type of food do you think your body will desperately want you to eat? You guessed it. Sugar. Almost nothing raises your blood glucose faster, and your biochemical drive for survival knows it. And now you feel so desperate for it, nothing is going to stand in your way. But if you give in and you eat something, when you said you wouldn't, what emotion do you feel? G-U-I-L-T. And what stress hormone do you think guilt drives your body to make? C-O-R-T-I-S-O-L. What a vicious cycle.

So you give in and you eat whatever sweet fix you can lay your hands on. Some women will placate the need for food at this time by having their second coffee of the day. There's no way a black coffee would hit the spot at this time of day, though. Because you are actually hungry you will typically choose a milk-based coffee here. Those who choose the coffee option feel mildly pleased because they didn't give in and eat—but then these people "know" in the back of their mind that a second coffee is not ideal for them either. New clients express precisely this to me every day of my working life. They console themselves with, "at least I didn't eat," but whether you choose the coffee or the food, your blood glucose will rise again, as will insulin. *And hello fat storage situation number four of the day.*

Then the self-directed, silent, cruel statements typically begin. "You are hopeless. You have no willpower. Look at your stomach." It is the "will I, won't I, I said I wouldn't, but I did" syndrome. And in that mindset, you are still at your desk at 6:30 p.m., still trying to get on top of the work you didn't do that day because you were so busy thinking about food and exercise and dresses and your stomach and not passing gas, that you *can't* go to the gym now because it is already 6:30 p.m. You still have more work to do, and if you work until 7:15 p.m., well, there's no food at home so you will have to go grocery shopping on your way home, but, if you do, it will be 8 p.m. before you get home and then you still have to chop the vegetables, and you feel like that takes ages. And then you still have to cook, eat, and clean up, so it will be at least 11:30 p.m. before you are finished doing all of that, and you probably need to do more work at home that night. But you have to wash your hair in the morning and then straighten it and you need to get up earlier to do that…

And then you get up and do it all over again, and you wonder why you can't lose weight when you don't eat "that badly." I know I used a similar scenario earlier in the stress hormones discussion, but it seemed appropriate here as well—and it is a pattern common to many, many women. I call it "Rushing Woman's Syndrome" (RWS for ease of expression; and it resonated so powerfully for so many women that I went on to write a book specifically about and titled *Rushing Woman's Syndrome*).

Although I may have exaggerated some of the details of the scenario above—or not really—and there are many variations to what I have described, which may include children, partners, parents, or friends, I meet women of all ages who live like this and also some men.

There may or may not be big, traumatic stresses going on, but there is a daily, relentless juggling act that never ends. Such a scenario is typical of adults aged between 25 and 65, although it tends to be far more prominent in those between 30 and 55. It comes from a desire to make others happy, from being a "pleaser" in your nature, behavior that was likely rewarded in childhood. You feel good helping out and being there for others, but you never, ever put yourself first. You are exhausted underneath your smile and, if you don't feel that way, you are usually living on adrenalin. I talked about this in my TEDx talk.

The cocktail of hormones being made in these scenarios mostly involves adrenalin, cortisol, and insulin. This disastrous cocktail in turn interferes with progesterone production, so estrogen becomes dominant. This down regulates thyroid function so you drink coffee or wine, or both, to warm up and cool down respectively each day—and, as a result, your liver gets a regular thumping. And still no one eats enough vegetables. Throw in some emotional confusion and chaos, still to be addressed, and you have *Accidentally Overweight*. Can you now see why I suggested earlier in this book that it is never about the food—but yet on the other hand, it is about the food? It's time to slow down, beautiful people.

How the biochemistry of insulin relates to appetite and fat storage

Please understand that I am not suggesting that we are not responsible for how much and what we eat. We are 100 percent responsible for this. Nor am I saying that willpower plays no role. Of course it can. My concern is that many people view food, weight, fat, and size simply as components of calories in versus calories burned equation, and they believe that if you eat anything other than what you know to be healthy, then you are useless. What I simply want to point out to the world is that our hormones are powerful, and your drive for safety and survival overrides everything.

Regardless of how frustrated you may be with your ever-expanding size, take the time to explore your whys. Which hormones identified in this book so far stand out to you? Do you think that you eat emotionally? Read on to learn more about the power and interrelationships of insulin.

Over the past 30 or so years what has become known as the "obesity epidemic" has unfolded. People tend to judge others and assume they must eat too much and move too little for them to be the size that they are, and there are times when this is accurate, but there are times when this is not. Judgment is explored on page 188 in Puzzle Piece 9, Emotions, and is one of unhealthiest emotions you can experience—for both the judger and the person being judged.

However, what I want to explore with you now is—what is it about the physiology of the human body that allows this to happen? Our biochemistry has what are called "built-in negative feedback mechanisms," which are supposed to stop us from gaining too much weight. In some people, this is not working efficiently or, if it is, it is being ignored biochemically. Scientists have been exploring what has the ability to block the signals telling our body to eat less and move more. Clearly, something is getting in the way. And most research indicates that insulin is precisely this block.[12] The entire role of insulin is to store energy for later and, in a world of plenty, in a world full of processed carbs—because insulin does its job—we gain weight.

As described earlier, insulin moves glucose out of the blood and into the muscles and fat cells, which results in weight increase. But regardless of size—although this scenario tends to be more distinct in very overweight people—if insulin levels are high, another hormone called leptin is supposed to kick in and tell your brain that you've eaten. Leptin is produced by fat cells, and circulates through the blood, binding to receptors in the hypothalamus, the area of the brain that controls energy balance.

Leptin is supposed to turn off the desire to eat. In addition to this, it also triggers the involvement of the autonomic nervous system—various parts of which either promote or block fat burning. Through research that involved suppressing insulin with a drug, it has been shown that insulin interferes with leptin's ability to signal to the brain to stop eating. However, studies in which leptin was given to obese people under the hypothesis that it would shut off appetite[13] have usually found that it is not the miracle pill it was anticipated to be, and here's why. It appears that insulin stops your brain from being able to "see" leptin, which leaves leptin lousy at down regulating appetite. The key here is that insulin must first come down for appetite to decrease, especially the desire for carbohydrates, and for weight loss to be sustained.

The importance of exercise

Resistance exercise is essential and the best "drug" of all for dealing with insulin. We are crazy if we think exercise only works by burning calories. Just 20 minutes of jogging equals one chocolate chip biscuit. One fast-food hamburger equals three hours of vigorous exercise to "work it off." The reasons behind the importance of exercise are far beyond burning calories.

First, exercise increases the sensitivity of skeletal muscle to insulin. When this happens your pancreas can make less insulin, so your levels of insulin will decrease. And the result will be less insulin required in your blood to move glucose into fat cells (after the liver and muscles stores are satisfied). In other words, less insulin means less glucose (sugar) being turned into fat.

The second reason that movement is important is because, after diaphragmatic breathing, certain types of exercise are the single best "treatments" to lower cortisol, your chronic stress hormone. More on this in a moment. Cortisol lays down what is known as "bad" visceral fat, the fat around the middle, stored so your body will always have energy to escape from danger (real or perceived) and to keep you alive. By reducing cortisol you are decreasing the amount of fat that gets deposited around your middle, and this also inadvertently reduces your food intake.

Fructose and the liver: Their relationship to insulin

An excess of any food or beverage over time can make you lay down additional body fat. But there are some that need to be looked at in more detail. One—fructose—is a dietary component well worth discussing when it comes to insulin.

Fructose is the carbohydrate found naturally in foods such as fruit, corn, and honey. The trouble is human consumption of fructose has significantly escalated over the past 30 years or so, as it has been added to more and more processed foods. Our bodies are simply not designed to consume so much of it. Most people (unless you are excluding fruit to see if it decreases your bloating) can handle two pieces of fruit per day and some honey in tea. There is usually no problem with this, except in specific health conditions, relating mainly to liver and/or gut health or an autoimmune condition. Fruit, honey, and corn themselves are nourishing foods. Please hear this. For most people, it is the *overconsumption* of fructose that is the problem. US statistics suggest that the consumption of fructose has increased from about 9oz (250g) per year in 1970 to 55lb (25kg) per year in 2003, an enormous escalation caused by a massive increase in the consumption of processed foods.

Originally, fructose was used in food products for people with diabetes; it has a low glycemic index (GI), meaning it is digested slowly so drives a very modest insulin response. Researchers had suggested that fructose was not actually regulated by insulin and, therefore, it was presented to the world as the "perfect sugar for people with diabetes." High fructose corn syrup (HFCS) came on the market after it was invented in 1966, and it began to find its way into US foods in 1975. In 1980, soft drink companies started to introduce it into soft drinks. Research suggests that the prevalence of childhood obesity in the USA can be traced back to this shift. Even though the chemistry of fat burning is multifaceted, widespread use of HFCS certainly hasn't helped and research suggests that it has added dramatically to the roadblocks to fat burning.

The difference with fructose is not the number of calories per gram. In this respect, it is no different from glucose. The biggest difference is that the only organ in your body that can actually take up fructose is your liver. The body cannot use fructose for energy; it must first be changed into glucose and an enzyme made by the liver makes is essential for this process. Every organ, on the other hand, can take up glucose, and only about 20 percent of your glucose load arrives at your liver. The fewer loads on the liver, the better! It is important to note, however, that sucrose (table sugar) is made up of glucose and fructose joined together, so sucrose also places an additional load on the liver particularly due to its fructose content, and sucrose is the predominant sweetener in foods in Australia, New Zealand, and the UK.

The excessive consumption of fructose has been shown to do three not so great things within the liver; in fact fructose has been shown to be a hepato-toxin ("hepato" meaning liver). First, it drives the liver to make additional uric acid, the accumulation of which causes gout. It has also been suggested that elevated uric acid is the basis of some forms of high blood pressure. Uric acid inhibits nitric oxide, which is one of the body's natural blood-pressure-lowering agents. Second, excess fructose consumption initiates what is called, in scientific circles, de novo lipogenesis, meaning "new fat synthesis," which can lead to problems with blood fats and the ratio of cholesterol and triglycerides (free fat) in the blood. And, third, it appears that excessive consumption of fructose can drive inflammation in the liver, which appears to stop the liver's insulin receptors from working effectively. When this happens, insulin levels throughout the entire body rise, so even though we link insulin to blood glucose and the pancreas—since that is where it is made—you can also see how blood sugar dysregulation and/or insulin resistance is related to liver function. I say it again: we must look after our liver! The effects of elevated insulin are actually systemic.

As you now know, when insulin levels rise, they tell every cell of your body to store fat, and they can interfere with normal brain metabolism of the insulin signal, which is linked to leptin (as described above). If you put all of this together, elevated insulin not only leads to increased body fat but also to increased fat in the liver and the liver driving more and more deposition of body fat as well as increased inflammation. My goodness! What you end up with is what has become known as a non-alcoholic fatty liver, which is now known as a disease.

When this is going on, your brain can't receive the signal from leptin to stop eating, so you consume more, and this is usually processed carbohydrates. What a vicious cycle! Imagine if you threw in a few alcoholic drinks each week on top of that chemical chaos! And so many people do. It is not surprising so many people feel lousy. In the USA, soft drinks and many processed foods, such as pretzels, contain high fructose corn syrup, which is either 42 or 55 percent fructose. In Australia, New Zealand and the UK, soft drinks and most of what I call "birthday party" foods contain sucrose. Sucrose (table sugars) is 50 percent fructose (the rest is glucose), so both are of great concern. Ouch, our liver!

Before you panic and go to a dietary extreme, as humans are so good at doing—sometimes to their long-term detriment—remind yourself that fructose, when combined with fiber, such as naturally occurs in fruit, is far better for us (obviously) than cakes, cookies, chocolate, and candy (sweets). For example, an average-sized orange has 20 calories, 10 of which are fructose, and it is high in fiber. A glass of orange juice has 126 calories. It takes six oranges to make that glass of juice, and it contains zero fiber. Dietary fiber is important because it slows the rate of intestinal carbohydrate absorption, which in itself reduces the insulin response.

Do your best to choose food as you would find it in nature. Don't be a fruit bat and eat eight pieces a day. Two is perfect or, as I said earlier, zero for a four-week trial to get on top of bloating or for specific health reasons. An experienced health professional will guide you if you need additional vitamin C or other nutrients in your diet without fruit.

If you have eliminated fruit and are reintroducing it, bring it back first on an empty stomach, and see how you tolerate it. Remember, one aspect of exploring your health is about giving you answers to pain, feelings of discomfort, or even illness in your body; four weeks of dietary changes may provide you with some insight. It is up to you to decide what you do with your new information. Truly caring about yourself is paramount, and Puzzle Piece 9, Emotions, will reveal a new way of doing this.

The glycemic index and glycemic load

The glycemic index (GI) is the response of your blood glucose to 50g of carbohydrate in that food. Discovery of the GI in 1981[14] gradually changed the face of treatment for Type 1 and Type 2 diabetes, which are in fact biochemically two very different conditions. A food can be classed as low GI because it makes your blood sugar rise very slowly, causing only a small amount of insulin (fat storage hormone) to be secreted. On the other hand, a carbohydrate that is digested quickly causes blood sugar to rise quickly, requiring insulin and hence fat storage signals to surge.

In my opinion and experience, the GI is a very small part of this picture. I prefer to talk about choosing foods that are low HI—low human intervention. Nature knows best. Furthermore, what is now known as the glycemic load (GL) has come to be shown as a far better guide when it comes to foods, if we need a guide other than nature, which I suggest we don't. Take carrots for example. Carrots are very high GI. If you eat 50g of carbohydrate in carrots (please note, that does not mean 50g total of carrots, it is referring to 50g of the carbohydrates in carrots, as they contain other substances such as fiber and water), your blood sugar goes up very high; hence it is a high-GI food. Fructose, on the other hand, has a low GI. Soft drinks in the USA have a GI of 53, which is low, but this is because they are based on high fructose corn syrup. If you only considered the GI, you would say carrots are bad for fat storage and soft drinks are fine, but of course common sense, nature, and, in this case, science must prevail. Enter the GL.

The GL is the GI multiplied by the amount of food you would actually have to eat to ingest the 50g of carbohydrate. So with carrots, you would have to eat an entire truckload to go close to eating 50g of carbohydrates from carrots. I've not met anyone who has done that, and I'm not suggesting you try! So even though carrots have a high GI, they have a low GL, whereas soft drinks have nothing going for them from a nutritional perspective and have a very high GL, despite having a low GI. Plus we now understand the impact excessive fructose has on the liver. Nature shows us we are supposed to eat our carbohydrates with fiber as this helps to lower the GL of the carbohydrate.

Or to keep it simple, which is always the best way with food… when it comes to food, nature gets it right. Use common sense. Choose low-GI food.

Sweetness of life

I hope it is clear that although this book is about solving your weight-loss puzzle, I am also gently unfolding information that might open your eyes and your heart to the concept that weight loss involves the superb interaction of many biochemical systems, and that your thoughts, beliefs, and perceptions are just as powerful, if not more powerful than the food you eat.

Louise Hay teaches that blood glucose is all about the sweetness we perceive in our life. In Type 2 diabetes or insulin resistance, when the blood sugar is elevated, she suggests that your perception of your life is that you have nothing to look forward to. If this resonates for you, I suggest you schedule things in your life that you love and start to notice the immense beauty around you. You can look forward to the surprise of what the sunrise will look like tomorrow.

Signs your blood glucose or insulin response needs support

- You crave sugars and/or starches. You really love carbohydrates

- You feel like you live on an energy rollercoaster and when you feel exhausted or bored, you go hunting for carbs (or caffeine)

- You eat processed foods

- You have Type 2 diabetes

- You have been diagnosed with "pre-diabetes (Type 2)" or insulin resistance

- You have a poor (low) muscle mass

- You focus more on exercise than dietary changes as a weight-loss strategy

- You live on adrenalin

- You feel like you run out of petrol in your energy tank if you go too long without carbs

- You feel like life is full of pressure and urgency

- You have skin tags

- Most days you warm up with caffeine and cool down with alcohol, and you eat processed foods in between

- You have been diagnosed with a fatty liver

- You have elevated blood cholesterol

- You have elevated blood triglycerides.

INSULIN SOLUTIONS

As I said earlier, I live in the same world as you with the same food on offer, and I want to offer practical solutions for you. However, I encourage you to be strict in the initial phases of change, partly to show you how good you can feel but also to break your habits. If you first need to increase your greens or whole-food fats before omitting sugar, then do that. And then cut it out for four weeks. No excuses.

- Eat food the way it comes in nature as often as you can.

  > Limit foods out of packets.

  > Limit refined sugar and foods that have had sugar added to them; after beautiful cane juice is squeezed out of sugar cane, the liquid is processed 14 times to create the white powder that you then eat. There is zero goodness in sugar.

  > Only eat completely natural carbohydrates for four weeks.

  > Eat lentils, root vegetables, berries, and other fruits, but keep fruit to two pieces a day maximum to reduce the requirement for insulin. Please note, this does not mean cut the carbs out. It means just what I said, which is don't eat carbs out of packets, and limit fruit to two pieces per day.

  > Limit alcohol, as it drives an enormous blood glucose surge and a rapid elevation of insulin.

  > If you do drink alcohol, consume it with food.

  > Many people are actually hungry and/or thirsty when they want a drink. Do an experiment. If it is the sugar (carbs) in the alcohol you want, eat a carrot or have a sparkling water in a wine glass with some fresh lemon or lime. Notice if the fizz from the water or the coldness of the drink helps quench your thirst.

  > Many people tell me that if they make it past the "witching hour" their desire for alcohol passes. Get some strategies to get past this time in your day.

> Have blood tests for blood glucose levels (BGL) and blood insulin.

- Eat five to six small meals per day—every three hours—if you are hungry and if this assists you to make better food choices, rather than waiting until you are ravenously hungry and craving poor-quality food. You will notice that the more fat from real food you include, the more satiated you will feel. As your metabolism starts to shift from relying solely on glucose as its fuel, to one of efficient fat burning, your hunger will decrease and you won't feel like you need to eat as frequently. This is a journey. I've had countless clients go from eating six times a day and struggling not to overeat, to eating two to three times a day and feeling very energized and satisfied.

- Eat whole-food fats with every meal. You may feel that eating protein with every meal serves your health.

- Build muscle with resistance training to help your muscles to remain highly insulin-sensitive, therefore requiring less insulin across your lifetime.

- Insulin is a growth factor and a fat storage hormone. Skin tags are a sign that your insulin was likely in excess at some (current or past) time.

- Cow's milk is made by cows to feed their young. It is created to grow an 90lb (40kg) calf into a 2,000lb (900kg) beast. Humans were never designed to grow at these rates. Limit or omit it, and, if you do consume it, only eat organic dairy.

- Apply the liver and adrenal support strategies (*see page 65 in Puzzle Piece 2, Stress Hormones, and page 117 in Puzzle Piece 4, The Liver*).

- Avoid artificial sweeteners, as we have no idea of their long-term effect on the human body. I pray they are safe as people consume masses of them these days. There is an enormous difference between exposing mice under test conditions to a substance for less than a year and humans consuming them for their entire lifetime. I am also suspicious that although they do not contain calories, they are confusing the insulin response. Some of the physically largest people I have ever met drank literally gallons of diet soft drinks every day, almost like an addiction. Leave it on the shelf. Use sparkling water with fresh fruit to sweeten the transition.

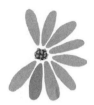

Puzzle Piece 8
The Nervous System

The focus of this piece of your weight-loss puzzle is the nervous system itself, and the way it contributes to the type of fuel the body believes it needs to use in order to best serve your health. And what you will see is that, as with other systems in the body, you are wired for survival. In modern times, however, this can disrupt the efficient utilization of body fat as a fuel.

The autonomic nervous system

Everything in our internal and external environments, including the food we eat, the exercise we do (or don't do), and the thoughts we think, influences our nervous system. Most people believe that in order to become healthy they must lose some weight. I believe the opposite is true; in order to lose weight, we must become healthy, and I approach weight loss for clients in this way.

As I've described, using science, emotion, and real-life stories throughout this book, I have known thousands of people who subsist on very little, and exercise frequently, but never get anywhere when it comes to fat loss. How else can we approach this? And how does this lifestyle create Rushing Woman's Syndrome? For some, RWS is at the heart of them becoming *Accidentally Overweight*.

Don't get me wrong. I meet women living the RWS life and they are slim. But their nervous systems are usually a wreck.

To understand this, we need to explore how the autonomic nervous system (ANS) works. The autonomic nervous system "runs" our body behind the scenes and it is not under our conscious control. It regulates our heart rate, respiration rate, temperature control, and immune and hormonal systems while we carry on with life. Don't you think it is truly miraculous that if you cut yourself the wound just heals? Don't you think it is amazing that you swallow food and your digestive system extracts the nutrients to nourish you so you can stay alive? The human body is extraordinary and that's an understatement.

There are three parts to the autonomic nervous system. They are the sympathetic nervous system (SNS), the parasympathetic nervous system (PNS), and the enteric nervous system (ENS). Here I will focus on the SNS, the "fight-or-flight" system, and the PNS, the "rest and repair" system, and their interaction.

In general, the SNS and the PNS have opposite functions. When we are under stress, the SNS (as discussed on page 61 in Puzzle Piece 2, Stress Hormones), raises our heart rate, increases our respiratory rate, releases cortisol and shunts blood away from the digestive tract to the muscles so that we can run away or fight whatever is threatening us. If organ systems in the body are unhealthy, and therefore stressed themselves, or if we are mentally or emotionally stressed, that increases the sympathetic load as well. The SNS by its very nature is catabolic, meaning that it breaks down muscle tissue due to the increased amounts of secreted cortisol. High-intensity exercise is also sympathetic in nature; the heart rate goes up, as do respiration and body temperature, and cortisol is released into the blood. And we know what cortisol does to body fat and the hormonal changes it initiates. Once the "threat' is dealt with (is it ever dealt with in the modern world?), the PNS slows our heart rate and respiration and it brings the blood back to the digestive tract so that we can digest our food. It also works on repairing any tissues that have been damaged in our "battle" and allows libido to be restored. Your survival instinct can't have you thinking about reproduction when your body believes that your life is being threatened.

The PNS is able to do its wonderful work overnight, provided we go to bed early enough, because cortisol naturally starts to rise around 2 a.m. The SNS and the PNS are designed to balance each other. In those people who have a well-balanced nervous system, high-intensity exercise tends to lead to fat loss because the parasympathetic rest time between workouts is when muscle tissue is built. High-intensity exercise has other metabolic and biochemical consequences; however, the scope of this book does not explore them.

It is likely that people who are unable to lose fat by doing regular high-intensity exercise have a dominant SNS and, as a result, an inhibited PNS. In situations like this, there is too much systemic stress coming from somewhere, therefore adding high-intensity exercise is counterproductive. It adds to an individual's sympathetic load, exacerbating the nervous system imbalance. This is one of the reasons we have to get our heads around "it's not about the calories." If "burning" more of them has not solved your body-fat challenge up until now, it is not suddenly going to start until some other work is done. And once the other work is done, you won't need to go back to sustained, high-intensity exercise and caloric deprivation to maintain your new level of health and the size and shape of your body.

Anxiety is so incredibly common today, often as a result of relationship challenges, financial stress, a poor diet and its consequences, worries about health or weight or if you've upset someone. Yet, a person may be in sympathetic overload and still not even mention feeling anxious.

Reducing the sympathetic load is essential to fat loss if the SNS is dominant. Movement is still important, but it is best approached from a different angle and with a different attitude. Far more effective exercise for SNS-dominant people is what I call the more "yin" (gentle, feminine, as opposed to "yang," masculine, go go go) exercise types such as tai chi, qi gong, yoga, Stillness Through Movement, or any exercise that is done slowly while being conscious of the breath. These types of exercise significantly assist in increasing PNS activity, which helps balance the ANS. Building muscle is also critically important to—among other things—metabolic rate, and long-duration high-intensity workouts tend to break muscle down, not build it. Once the nervous system is better balanced, body fat is readily burned, a concept that is game-changing to the way you approach your body and your health.

The nervous system and body fat

In any given moment the human body is making a decision about which fuel to use based on the information it is receiving from the internal and external environments. The only two fuels for the human body are glucose (sugar) and fat. You don't use protein for fuel. The body breaks proteins down into amino acids, which are then converted into glucose so the body can use that glucose as fuel (energy). The name of this biochemical pathway is "gluconeogenesis." The body requires energy for everything it does, from walking to sleeping, laughing to blinking; it all requires fuel.

As you now know, adrenalin communicates to every cell of your body that your life is in danger and it prepares you to fight or flee. However, you may be making adrenalin simply because you have to make a phone call that you'd rather not make or perhaps because you've gulped down three coffees already today. Or maybe your dad yelled at you a lot when you were a child and so even though you know now that your dad yelled a lot because that was how he communicated and coped with how stressed he felt (rather than it being about his lack of love for you), now when a male in your life raises his voice in your vicinity, you instinctively go into the "fight-or-flight" response. The majority of stress for most people in the Western world today is psychological rather than physical and it can be constant and relentless.

The branch of the nervous system that is activated with stress of any type is the SNS, which has an intimate relationship with adrenalin. If the body's perception is that it needs to escape from impending danger, whether your thinking mind is telling you so or not, you need a fast-burning fuel available to you to do that. Your body thinks it has to get out of there and get out of there fast! So what fuel do you think your body will choose when it needs to flee, to get out of "danger" fast? Remember its only choice is to burn either sugar or fat... in this scenario, it will choose sugar every time. The body thinks it has to in order to save our life and we are all about survival. The body doesn't feel "safe" enough to use fat as its fuel in this "fight-or-flight" state because fat offers us a steady, slow-release form of energy—not what we need in a time of danger. We can burn fat effectively in a PNS-dominant state because the body perceives it is safe when the PNS is activated. Yet, the PNS can never be the dominant arm of the ANS, it can never steer the ship, while the body perceives there may be a threat to your life. This alone can be a significant block to utilizing body fat as a fuel and therefore weight loss.

We have glucose stored in our muscles and liver in a form called glycogen, and these stores are mobilized whenever our body gets the message that it needs energy to fight or run, if there is not enough glucose to fuel our escape left in our blood from our last meal. This mobilization of glycogen out of the muscles due to stress can, over time, impact the function and appearance of our muscles, including allowing the onset of cellulite.

I believe that one of the most enormous health challenges of modern times is that the body can constantly be on the receiving end of the "fight-or-flight" messages. There are so many factors, internal and external to us, which drive this response within us that we have to begin to choose actively not to go there, not to get caught up in the rush. And to take steps in our daily lives to allow our nervous system to have some balance. Without this, using fat as a fuel can be an uphill battle.

Craving sugar

Many people today know they need to eat less sugar or cut it out completely. You would have to have had your head buried in the sand not to know that eating refined sugars does not serve your health in any way. Yet, even with great understanding of this topic and even with the desire to change dietary sugar habits, many people describe it being the major challenge for them on their road to outstanding health. So why is it that we crave sugar so much?

One reason is certainly habit. Another is its infiltration into the food supply, even into savory-tasting foods, and taste preference for sweeter and sweeter foods is also playing a role. It is a case of more begets more. Very few people go back after dinner for a second helping of broccoli. Yet what most people are not familiar with is the impact of the biochemistry, of stress hormone production on sugar cravings.

As you now understand, there are only two fuels for the human body: glucose and fat. And when you are living on stress hormones because of too much caffeine or due to your perception of pressure and urgency, your body predominantly uses glucose as its fuel, not body fat. A person weighing 155lb (70kg) has the capacity to store about 2,500 calories of glucose (as glycogen in their liver and muscles) while that same person will store about 130,000 calories of fat. So the more your body thinks it needs to use glucose as your fuel to help you escape from danger, the more it needs to keep your "get out of danger" fuel tank full. So you crave it to support yet another survival mechanism.

Too many people in the Western world today regularly over consume caffeine, feel pressured about their work, money, relationships or their body, feel like all of their tasks are urgent, like there aren't enough hours in the day and they scratch the itch of their "not enoughness" (*explored further on page 186 in Puzzle Piece 9, Emotions*) on and off all day. Then they crave wine in the evenings for the sugar and to help them relax, even though underneath they are utterly exhausted. And many people have become so accustomed to living this way, they don't even notice how stressed they are anymore. Anxiety is rife, yet most people who experience it have not been informed that caffeine leads them to make the very hormone that drives anxious feelings. If you experience such feelings, caffeine needs to be the first thing that goes.

When you live like this, your body will predominantly use glucose as a fuel in preference to body fat and it will only switch back to being an efficient fat burner if you make some changes. You can start with the food—some people do—yet for others starting here is precisely why they've made no progress in decreasing or cutting refined sugars and refined starches out (remember both sugars and starches are all broken down to glucose in the digestive system).

So if you know starting with food is not your way, then park it. You can start by focusing on activating your PNS, which means embracing diaphragmatic breathing. This may take the form of a restorative, breath-focused practice such as restorative yoga, tai chi, meditation, or simply regular intervals across the day where you commit to 20 long, slow breaths that move your belly as you breathe. It is a matter of retraining yourself to breathe this way, instead of the short, sharp, shallow breaths in your upper chest that adrenalin drives. The calmer you feel, the more your PNS is activated, the less sugar your *body* will need to keep the glucose fuel tank full.

Increasing your intake of green vegetables and/or dietary fats from whole-food sources can also make a big difference in reducing your desire for sugar. A high intake of green leafy vegetables for a minimum of 21 days starts to change your taste preferences, as greens have a bitter taste base. When it comes to fat, if you've lived through the "low fat, high carb" era and you became conscious of your dietary fat intake, you may not be eating enough of it. Notice when you crave sugar and significantly increase your intake of fats at the meal prior to the typical craving time. For example, if the middle of the afternoon is your tough time, then eat more whole-food fat at lunchtime.

Fat is incredibly satiating and you'll notice it will fuel you for longer through your afternoon. Yet if you still have the mindset that counting calories is your only road to weight loss, you'll never let yourself eat the fat, given it has the highest number of calories per gram. However, when you eat carbohydrates it leads the body to make insulin, which you now understand signals to the body to store fat, whereas when you eat dietary fat, no fat-storage signaling hormones are released. Not all calories behave equally *inside* the body, a concept I explore in detail in my book *The Calorie Fallacy*.

Signs your nervous system needs support

- You feel stressed regularly and like you are on red alert

- No matter how well you count calories and exercise, you struggle to lose weight (I'm not suggesting you count calories, but rather that you use this as a sign that this puzzle piece may need to be addressed)

- You crave sugars and/or starches (carbohydrates)

- You love coffee, energy drinks, and anything that contains caffeine, although sometimes you notice that they make your heart race

- You startle (jump) easily

- You regularly don't sleep well

- You don't wake up restored or with good energy

- If you don't go to sleep by 10 p.m., you get a second wind and end up staying awake until at least 1 a.m.

- You regularly feel tired but wired

- You are a worrier or a drama queen (or king)

- You feel anxious easily

- Your breathing tends to be shallow and quite fast

- You experience "air hunger" (and other causes have been ruled out)

- You struggle to say "No"

- You laugh less than you used to

- You feel like everything is urgent

- You feel like there aren't enough hours in the day.

NERVOUS SYSTEM SOLUTIONS

When you understand how your nervous system works then you start to see what it needs, and I hope the following solutions will help you put that information to good use.

- Embrace a restorative practice.

- Commit to a regular practice of diaphragmatic breathing.

- Instead of focusing on eating less sugar, focus on eating more dietary fats from whole foods and/or green vegetables.

- Decrease or omit caffeine for four weeks (and keep it going if it feels much calmer), or switch from coffee to green tea so that you consume smaller amounts of caffeine buffered by the effects of theanine in the green tea.

- Explore your perception of pressure and urgency. Have you made what you have to do each day full of pressure and urgency? Or is it a busy life, full of opportunity that is so ridiculously privileged because all of your basic needs are met? Of course there is real pressure and real urgency in this world. But save that perception for when you really need it, not your everyday existence (explored in detail in my book *Rushing Woman's Syndrome*).

- Explore your emotional landscape using the strategies in the next chapter, Emotions, if feeling like you are not good enough resonates for you.

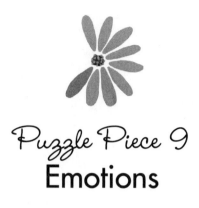

Puzzle Piece 9
Emotions

Most of us know what to eat; we just don't do it. Even with all the confusing nutrition information out there—such as "eat carbs as they are essential for energy" versus "don't eat carbs because they will make you fat and tired"—and these statements can be made in books sitting right beside one another on the same bookshelf—most of us still have a general idea about the food that nourishes us. And we still don't do it. And this is not just about food and body size. I have met plenty of slim people who are incredibly unhealthy. Just because it might not show on the outside doesn't mean you've got this piece of the puzzle licked. Most of us know it is not great to drink bucketloads of alcohol or caffeine, for example, either, yet at times we still do.

If food, certain beverages, your body, or your weight are areas that you struggle with and argue about in your mind, you can spend your life in search of the right diet or the magic bullet or a time in your life when you are not so stressed and will finally be able to focus on your health. These things never come of their own accord. We always plan to do it tomorrow.

Since you already know *how* to eat and drink, my words are simply to remind you of what you already know. Some of you may not actually want to hear it even though you tell yourself you'd do anything for better health, a slimmer body, or both. Nature gets it right when it comes to food. So mostly choose these foods. Sure, there can be areas where you might need some guidance for a specific health picture, such as estrogen dominance, anxiety, food intolerances, or insulin resistance. And that is certainly what health professionals are for. And if you are confused about what to eat, then we guide you with that, too. In fact, I always guide people with the practicalities of solving estrogen dominance, anxiety, food intolerances or insulin resistance (for example), so they can start achieving results and also because these changes can be a stepping-stone to the emotions we actually need to explore.

Some emotions don't surface until you start going without what has been your numbing device: too many sweet foods, bread, coffee, and alcohol. What I am saying is that if you are physically too big for optimal health, then it is usually not a lack of knowledge that got you there. It is not a lack of education that leads you to polish off an entire packet of chocolate cookies. It is biochemical or emotional or both. If it were as simple as applying what you know, then you would have lost weight years ago. In fact, you would never have put it on in the first place. So the question is, why don't you eat in a way that makes you feel your best? Why? And, as I said, this is not just about body size. It can be just as much about body symptoms such as reflux, sinus congestion, or diarrhea. If you eat or drink something, while in your heart you know it gives you reflux, blocked sinuses, or loose stools, what are you communicating to your body? You're saying, "I'm not listening."

Why do we do it? In my opinion, there will be a range of reasons, but they virtually all lead back to the same statement you are subconsciously telling yourself, "I don't really care about you." And why don't you care about yourself? Why will you do more for others than yourself? One reason may be that you live in the cloud of false belief that you are not enough the way you are. Eating in a way that doesn't serve you is a way to distance yourself from how things are when they are not how you want them to be.

The first way to begin to explore an emotional approach to eating is to go digging for what food means to you. The second way is about cognitively understanding your emotional landscape and the meanings and rules that you touch on regularly that fuel your life. The third is through the examination and the application of the principles and processes of your Em-Matrix ("Em" stands for emotional)—your emotional patterns. There is so much gold right here.

Food is...

As I outlined in the Calories piece of the puzzle, one of the first exercises I do at my weekend events with my clients when they want to get to the heart of why they overeat (or over consume alcohol, although we will focus on food here), is to ask them to complete the following sentence with the first word that flies into their head, no censorship.

I say, "Food is..." and they respond: "Yummy," "Delicious," "A pain in the neck," "Life," "Love," "My whole world," "Comfort," "Amazing." These are all words that quickly and easily fly out of people's mouths. For someone who has gained and lost the same 45–110lb (20–50kg) over the years, food frequently falls into the "pleasure" category. If I am going to guide someone to change the way they eat, and food is their biggest source of pleasure in life, if I don't delve into what else this person finds pleasurable and point this out and encourage them to experience more of this in their lives (such as connecting with the beauty of nature, their faith, or how playful their puppy is), the food changes will be temporary. Food either needs a new meaning, such as nourishment, or energy, or the other pleasure factors need amping-up in this person's life. Even just being aware of what food means to you is a great first step.

Case Study

One of my favorite examples to share about how this simple process changed a client's after-dinner food frenzy comes from a precious lady for whom food was mostly comfort. Julie had experienced huge emotional trauma, and, afterward, food had become her friend, her sweetness, and her joy in life. When she came to see me, she said she was so desperate to lose the weight, she believed it had affected her work, as her job was in the public spotlight and she was embarrassed by her growing size. When I did the "Food is..." exercise with her, it become clear that what she wanted was comfort.

I asked her how else she might find comfort in a way that did not involve food. She had spoken about how much she treasured her beloved, young daughters, and from her descriptions they sounded very sweet. I felt that when she ate in the evenings what she really wanted was a hug, to be comforted emotionally by another human, or by something bigger (in a spiritual sense), rather than by food. I asked her if she ever stood at the door of her girls' bedrooms and watched them sleeping. Tears immediately sprang to Julie's eyes. As Mark Twain said, "Any emotion if it is sincere, is involuntary," so I immediately knew this was meaningful to her. I suggested that, each evening after the girls had gone to bed, Julie complete her usual evening rituals in the kitchen and, instead of going straight to the refrigerator and then into the lounge for a private sweet feast and the TV, she go to her girls and watch them sleeping. I suggested she notice their breathing, the little lights in their rooms, their innocence, the delicate smell of their hair, and the way their arms poked out from beneath the covers. I invited her to take comfort from their presence in her life. I reminded her that she created them and that, for now, if the only way I could get her to appreciate how truly amazing she was, was by focusing on the little girls she had brought into this world, then that would be the best "medicine" in the world for her.

We both cried, and Julie knew with conviction that she had her perfect answer. After just four weeks of practice, her weight had fallen, and she had not even heard the call of sweet food. She had sweetness in spades watching her children sleep.

. . . .

Another point worthy of mention is that of food waste. So many people eat too much food because they don't want to waste it, a behavior that is often derived from childhood experiences. A client once told me that she had chickens in her backyard so she could give all of her leftovers to them. That was how she "managed" her challenge with throwing food out. For some, it simply takes a change of perception: Whether you throw it out or you overeat, either way it is a waste.

Understand your meanings and rules: The fuel for your life

Humans store fat when they do not feel safe, whatever that means to them. I don't necessarily mean safe from burglary, but rather psychologically safe. On a physical level, I can relate such fat storage back to cortisol and the many downstream effects of this catabolic, metabolism-slowing hormone. Yet to crack that cortisol challenge, emotions hold the true key.

Each of us have rules about what it means for us to feel safe—typically in the areas of relationships, finance, and work—as a result of the life experiences we have had to date. Trouble is, we don't usually know what these rules are. The life experiences to which I am referring don't have to be traumatic. Not in the slightest. What I am referring to are all of the experiences of your life, traumatic or not, that have shaped your personality, your bank balance, your relationships, your responses, and your body size, to name just a few.

Everyone creates explanations about what things mean based on their own experiences in life so far. They are created from the interactions we had as children with the adults around us. As adults, we continue to replay these same meanings, only we are not aware we are doing it. All we know is that we seem to react to people and what they say, or they always seem to react to us in what seems like an unpredictable or inappropriate way, or we forever find ourselves in conflict with certain people. It's like an itch that constantly gets scratched. You are often unaware that this is what's behind so much struggle or suffering in your life (and also the good stuff when the meanings serve you), including your relationship with food, your body, with alcohol, or with your partner. There are some meanings that serve us and some that no longer do. Some are simply outdated protection mechanisms that were set up because of experiences earlier in your life. And where once they might have kept you safe, now they simply hold you back.

The meanings and rules to which I am referring were (and still are being) written by your subconscious mind, the part of your brain that makes your heart beat and your hair grow without you having to tell them to do so. This part of your nervous system is estimated to process two to four million pieces of information per second, while your conscious mind only (!) processes around 134 pieces of information per second. Think about that. I mean, *really* think about that. Your subconscious is extremely powerful.

Specific meanings and rules

The psychology of eating is a fascinating area. In every person, there are emotions that, although we don't realize it, are incredibly painful for us to feel. These are typically rejection, failure, and guilt.

There are many more, but for simplicity's sake I will keep it to these three. All three may be a factor for someone, but there is almost always one that stands out. Many women, for example, are what I endearingly call "love bugs." Although men also, of course, find rejection painful, as adults the fear of feeling this emotion is often buried under another emotion they fear such as failure. Ouch!

A love bug functions between two polarities every day: love and rejection. Replace the word "love" with "connection" or "appreciation," if that helps you relate to this idea, but I'll keep using "love" to keep it simple. Without realizing it, we behave as if we want a life jam-packed with love—caring for others and ourselves, feeling appreciated and understood, living without conflict, the list is almost endless. Yet psychology 101 teaches us that humans will do more to avoid pain than they will ever do to have pleasure. So instead of behaving in a way that drives a life of love, we spend our lives trying to avoid rejection… and those two lives look very different.

Based on our life experiences, we have rules in our subconscious minds about what has to happen for us to feel love and rules about what has to happen for us to feel rejected. Most of us make it really easy for ourselves to feel the emotion we actually want to avoid—in this case—rejection. Simultaneously, our rules around love make it really hard for us to feel it easily or constantly. An example that has brought tears to countless women's eyes during a session is this one.

You drop your son at the school gate and catch the eye of another mum you have previously noticed and admired. For the first time, you have a lovely chat and although there may be no conscious thought about this event lifting your spirits, you carry on happily with your day. But that afternoon, when you collect your son from school, your new acquaintance doesn't speak to you. You feel like she snubs you. She looks straight through you. You wonder what you've done wrong. Did you offend her? Did you embarrass yourself? Did you mistake her interest in you when really she just had no one better to talk to? Did she only speak to you because not many other mums were around that morning? Are you not dressed well enough for her to connect with you this afternoon in front of others? You think to yourself that you've never fitted in with that crowd—with those types of women—anyway. Isn't it exhausting what we put ourselves through?

What you've actually touched on in this moment is what I have come to call your "not enoughness," an inkling—or a gaping wound—that you are not good enough; not OK the way you are. And for the millionth time in your life, you scratch this itch. Unfortunately, you don't realize that this is what you're doing—and what you have probably done many times in the past. All you know is that now you feel sad or irritated. You may start focusing on how big your thighs look in your jeans (not thin enough) or how you haven't phoned your sister for weeks (not a good enough sister) or other negative self-talk. And you might decide you want some wine or some food that doesn't really benefit you. As soon as you have even had this thought, you feel a little bit better because now you have something to look forward to and you've shifted your focus from your perception of your not enoughness to something that brings you pleasure. All you are doing is attempting to escape emotional pain.

Again, it's unlikely that you will consciously make the connection between your new acquaintance at the school gate, your "I'm not good enough" button, and your mood, but rather than easing through your afternoon, you feel flat and frustrated. Or perhaps you are simply in a bad mood, despite looking forward to your cake, your crackers, or your wine—or all of the above—when your morning had been rather delightful or at least not emotionally eventful. Yet who is usually on the receiving end of your sullen or irritated mood? Most often, without thinking, you direct it toward yourself and also the people you love the most in this world.

Of course it's obvious, you tell yourself, that your new acquaintance is too embarrassed to speak to you when certain other mothers are around because you've gained weight this year. So, just to prove to yourself that you really aren't good enough, you eat. Without realizing it, you want to escape the emotional pain of feeling like you are not enough—and therefore won't be loved—and prove yourself right; that you are, indeed, useless and have no willpower. No wonder you are fat, you tell yourself; that must be why people don't like you and your mother/father told you that you were an embarrassment.

And it was actually way back then, starting with some throwaway comment your mother or father made, when you first felt "not good enough." Not that they meant to hurt your feelings. As adults we consciously know that the way someone behaves is a reflection of them, not you, but your conscious mind isn't running your life in these moments. In fact you can't see any of this when you are in the throes of inhaling a box of crackers, half a block of cheese, and a few glasses of white wine…

As for your own family, or whoever else is on the receiving end of your change in mood, they don't understand why you are quiet or why you are overreacting to things that didn't bother you yesterday, or what they seem to have done wrong. Of course they haven't done anything. The bottom line is you feel rejected by your new acquaintance.

Through food and/or wine, you have simply escaped from the "pain," from the deep, human, primal fear that you are not good enough and therefore you won't be loved. And built in to the autonomic nervous system of a baby human is the belief that love is essential to your survival—because it is. You can't obtain your own food, clothing and shelter. Yet as adults, we know that a life with love in it is delicious, but we can also survive without it, as we can find our own food, clothing and shelter. Yet the vast majority of adults still live their lives as if love is essential to their survival. So when they scratch the itch of their not enoughness, the fear that they won't be loved is triggered and to an adult brain and heart that has never explored this, that leads you to feel as if your life itself is under threat. So to escape from your pain, you eat or drink too much or engage in some other activity to distract yourself.

What if I told you that your acquaintance at the school gate didn't see you that afternoon or she didn't register seeing you? You will tell me that you *saw* her see you. I will then suggest you ask yourself what many have found to be a life-changing question… "I wonder what might be going on for her?" We react to situations as if life revolves around us, as if every person's response or reaction is about us. That's how children are: egocentric. Don't take offense at the word "egocentric." It simply means that you believe that others are the way they are because of you. From an emotional maturation perspective, children are supposed to be egocentric. But we are supposed to evolve emotionally over time yet we aren't really taught strategies to do this, so too many people don't catch a glimpse of what is really at the heart of their overeating, or the other ways we employ to escape from emotional pain.

When we enquire within ourselves and wonder what might be going on for another person it opens us to insights and connection, rather than judgment and separation. Do you know what it is like to be her? How do you know that she doesn't have a million things to do before she gets home, where she has to make sure the house is perfect and the children are bathed and fed so that when her husband arrives home he won't raise his voice and tell her that she is useless and does nothing all day? What if a raised voice is *her* ultimate pain because her mother or father told her the same thing in the same way?

Her perceived "snub" had nothing to do with you and, whatever her story, her "snub" speaks volumes about her; her pain, her attitudes, her losses, her fears, her inattention, her loss of presence in that moment, her focus on her child, her to-do list… Love bugs need to ask, "I wonder what might be going on for them" quite regularly, until they can stop the daggers of "rejection" from penetrating their hearts.

I had a client for whom this question changed not just her life but her body, and I will never forget the glee on her face when she told me it had freed her from what she called "agony," which involved secret eating after dinner and awful self-talk as a consequence. She literally looked as though years had come off her face just from this new understanding.

If love bugs find themselves standing at the refrigerator, peering in as if the meaning of life must be contained inside, another useful question to ask themselves is, "What do I really want?" At first, your brain will probably tell you that of course you simply want chocolate or cookies, but if you keep asking yourself this question the veil will start to lift, and you will see that what you actually want is a hug or company or for someone to thank you for making their bed every day for the last 25 years. Yet it is not even about these things that you have now identified. It is about how you perceive having these things will make you *feel*. We are governed by how we feel. So the next question is, how will having a hug, or company, or a thank you make you feel? And your answer might be "appreciated" or "connected" or "comforted" or "loved." It is the *emotion* you are chasing, not the biscuits and not the hug. It is the feeling you are seeking. So then ask yourself, how else can you experience this emotion without it harming your health? And then do that. Or be that. Or schedule that.

Emotional pain can serve you

The belief that to feel emotional pain is too traumatic to bear is like looking at the world through the eyes of a child. As infants, if we didn't have love, attention, and someone to feed us, we would die. So when we are born, a powerful belief is born as well: Without love, we will die. The thing is, of course, while a child might perish without love, adults physically will not. Love is delicious, yes, but we won't die without it. The trouble is, if you "touch" this belief too easily because your subconscious mind is set up to do so, then your desire to escape from emotions you won't let yourself feel, let alone recognize, can be a constant and overwhelming battle.

To escape, some people choose food; some people drink two bottles of wine every night, while others chain-smoke a pack of cigarettes each day. Some exercise like they are possessed. Some people starve themselves. Some people eat. And every time you do this, you miss out on feeling what is really there. It is the desire to avoid this "pain," that makes you bolt. You bolt to the refrigerator, and you bolt from yourself and what you truly feel in that moment. Your way back home to yourself—and away from the fridge or whatever escape mechanism you use—lies in acknowledging the pain and truly experiencing that it will not kill you. If you feel sad, you feel sad. If you overeat regularly to blanket the sadness, you just give yourself an additional reason to be sad. Eating does not get rid of the sadness. It adds to it. Why not then simply acknowledge that you feel sad rather than escaping from your pain through food?

Let's break this down into a strategy you can work on. The first step is to recognize an emotion that is very tough for you to feel, whether it's rejection, failure, or guilt, and then explore what has to happen for you to feel this emotion. You will see that humans make it really easy to feel emotions that we perceive will bring us the most pain and that we therefore most want to avoid. Unless you have previously done some work in this area, the emotion you first want to work with was (more than likely) created from an experience you had when you were probably quite young.

Case Study

One of the most simple, yet transformational processes I have ever witnessed was Mrs. M, who came to see me for weight loss but said as soon as she arrived, "I eat too much cake after dinner every night. And if your only solution for my weight loss is to tell me to stop eating the cake, if it were that

*simple, I would have done it for myself already." So many
people feel this way.*

*So here was dear Mrs. M, a short-in-stature, 60-year-old
lady of Irish heritage. I asked her my millions of questions,
including ones about sinus congestion, if she used her bowels
every day and what her transition into menopause was like.
Then, as I do with all of my clients, I asked her if her parents
were still alive. When I ask that question, most people think
I am seeking their family history—looking for degenerative
diseases, such as heart disease, for example—and I am
partly doing that. But mostly I am watching and feeling for
their reaction to having their parents mentioned. In the case of
Mrs. M, it was very obvious that there were painful memories.
She shared that her mother had died while giving birth to
her and that her father hadn't spoken to her since she was
14 years old.*

*She went on to share, "My father brought me home from
the hospital to our large farm, which was in the middle of
nowhere in Ireland. I had four older brothers and the nearest
to me in age was 13. I grew up there. It was quiet but I liked
it and I was good at school and helped with the house. But
then when I was 14 my father wrote a letter of introduction
to an aunt and then put me on a boat to New Zealand to
live with her and I never heard from him again. He loved my
brothers enough to keep them, but he didn't love me enough
to keep me."*

*There in her history was what she was distancing herself from
with the cake—she believed that her father had loved her
brothers enough to keep them, but not her. Not that she sat on
the lounge each night saying to herself that her father didn't
love her—there was no awareness of the father scenario
while eating the cake—but there was her underlying belief in
her story. And I've seen it time and time again. Perceiving that*

a parent didn't love you is one of the commonest emotional reasons for poor-quality food behaviors.

But I believe everyone has a beautiful heart. Their behavior may be "challenging" at times but I questioned her perception of his lack of love for her. And so I said, "What if the opposite was true? What if your father loved you so much, his one and only daughter, the daughter his beloved wife died giving birth to, the daughter who was good at school, and who at 14 was probably about to start menstruating—and as he was an already relatively elderly father by this stage in her life, he most likely had no idea how he would support you through menarche? What if he loved you so much that he was prepared to send you away and never see you again to give you the best opportunity with your education and your life?"

She replied that she'd never considered that. I continued, "Well, you said your father is still alive. Do you have any way of contacting him?" She said she could probably get a phone number for him. I asked her if she would do that and then phone him and ask him why he had sent her away. And she said she would.

To my utter astonishment, this extraordinary lady phoned her father—to whom she hadn't spoken for 46 years—and asked him why he'd sent her away. He told her, among many other heartfelt reasons, that he loved her very much and wanted her to have a better life than he thought he could ever give her on the farm.

I didn't talk to Mrs. M about cake. She just stopped eating it. Well, after dinner every night, anyway. She still had the odd piece when she saw her friends for a cup of tea. And yes, she lost weight. But she said she didn't even mind now, although she was pleased. She just felt so happy. Yet she never would have been able to tell me that she had had an ache in her heart—an immense sadness—about her father, prior to our consultations. She just didn't understand why, when she knew how she needed to eat for good health, she didn't do it. She was simply distancing herself from how she perceived things were because they weren't how she wanted them to be.

* * * * * * * * * * * * * * * * * * *

Case Study

I'll give you another simple example to get you thinking. One of the first people I ever worked with was a publicly well-known woman who was "larger than life" (I'll call her Mary). Mary was gregarious, hilarious, likeable, financially successful and, as a result, very charitable. She arrived to see me with a statement that went something like "I've heard you do weight loss differently and, honey, I've tried everything." Mary went on to tell me that she felt "successful" in every area of her life except when it came to her body. She never mentioned "health." In everything she said, it was always about her size and weight; until I asked, she never mentioned her reflux, the trouble she had breathing, the regular headaches, or the eczema that had been present since childhood. "Health" was not on her radar. It's very useful to start noticing your language patterns because a great deal can be revealed through what you say and also what you don't say.

The other thing I noticed was the way Mary spoke about her mother. Her mother hadn't just irritated her; Mary despised her. She spoke about her in the present tense, so I was stunned to learn that her mother had actually passed away almost 20 years before. When I asked Mary if there was a time in her life when she could recall her relationship with her mother not being so diabolical, she said yes. If someone can recall when a relationship changed, it usually means (in their mind at least) that "something" has happened and that's where the exploration needs to begin.

Mary thought the direction I was taking in our session was a "load of rubbish," particularly as she'd already done years of therapy around her hatred for her mother. She paid lip service to the concept that her mother had done her best, but when she finished that statement with "blah, blah, blah," a roll of her eyes, and a wave of her hand, I knew her heart didn't believe it. So I delved deeper. After all, she'd ask me to help her be as "successful" with her weight as she was in other areas of her life.

I asked Mary to remember a time when things were dreadful between her and her mother and then also a time when it had felt fine, or even quite good, to be around her mother. She said she could remember both. Then I asked her to remember the day it changed. And for the first time, her face lost its intensity and tightness. When Mary was four years old, she had been playing outside by herself, not far from the house on the family farm. She fell and cut her eye, screaming out as she did so. Her mother came running from the house and shouted, "You should be more careful, and then you wouldn't get hurt."

In that moment, my client could have created any of the following meanings:

- *My mother loves me so much she wants to protect me from further injury/pain (love).*

- *Hooray! I got Mom's attention (success).*

- *I've disappointed my mother (guilt).*

- *My mother hates me and doesn't love me (rejection).*

- *My mother thinks I'm a failure (failure).*

Before we move on, contemplate why you think the mother responded this way. Could her thoughts have been:

- *My precious baby has fallen and hurt herself for the first time! I must warn her to be more careful so she doesn't get hurt again (love).*

- *I feel so guilty that I wasn't there to protect my baby girl (her own guilt).*

- *I am so useless because my baby has hurt herself (failure).*

You can see from the outside looking in to the situation that the mother's response to her child's accident came from a place of love and protection, and initially fear at how badly the child was injured. But for Mary it was the first time her mother raised her voice with her and she had now linked it to physical pain. Welcome to the beginning of a new "meaning" locked into your nervous system. This is how the "itch" I describe gets set up for constant scratching as you go through life.

The mother's delivery may have been rough or harsh or loud, but the intention was beautiful. Yet when I asked Mary what she thought her mother meant from the words she had spoken, she told me she was a "cruel, cruel woman who hated me." In that moment, when she was four, Mary created a meaning that her mother didn't love her. In her eyes, "how could anyone who loves you shout at you when you're hurt?"

That moment set up further challenging interactions between Mary and her mother. Why? Because, subconsciously she started looking for evidence of what she had begun to assume about herself.

Please note

These words are not intended to elicit any feelings of guilt for parents. Please keep in mind that creating meanings from what others say is part of being human (everyone does it), and yes, it shapes us, and who we become, but it also gives us the opportunity to learn and grow and contribute. The skill, growth and freedom comes with being able to step back and see the "story" you are telling yourself. If all of our needs were always met—in our own eyes—we would never contribute.

Think about it and you'll see evidence of this type of scenario everywhere. For example, you might be seven years old now and you are leaving the house for school, and your mother calls out, in a frustrated voice because she has 80,000 things to do that day and is running late, "It's cold outside and you've forgotten your sweater. Go and get your sweater." If you were Mary in this situation, and had in that first instance when you fell, created a meaning of "Wow, my mum loves me so much she never wants me to go through this pain again" (love), then when your mother reminds you to get your sweater, you would have skipped off to your room, grabbed your sweater, and happily gone off to school, regardless of the tone in her voice. In fact, you probably wouldn't even have noticed her "tone."

If, however, from that first instance, you created a meaning of rejection or failure, you would create that meaning again now from your mother's words reminding you to take your sweater to school, and you would validate that meaning by thinking to yourself, "See, she doesn't even think I can dress myself." You will stomp off to your room, collect your sweater, and go sullenly to school, only to have your mood lighten once you arrive and see your friends.

Can you see how two completely different lives could play out just from that one meaning, and therefore belief, that was created so early?

When you are little, from a psychological development perspective, you are the center of the universe. It is all about you. It has to be or you wouldn't survive, remember. But once you are older and have the opportunity to see such situations as if you are hovering above them, that clarity can be enough to elicit the most beautiful "healing," the most magnificent "a-ha" moments. When an adult "sees" a mistaken belief from childhood, the forgiveness and compassion for their parent's life, as well as a newfound compassion for themselves, are palpable and always an honor to witness.

It is important to acknowledge that the meanings we've created will have served us in some ways until now. Indeed, they may not have always brought you challenges. Until now, some of the meanings you have created will have done some great things for you. For example, if you were a part of the scenario above and the initial meaning you created was guilt, then you may have spent your life pleasing everyone so that you never felt like you were letting anyone down, and as a result people probably deeply love and appreciate you. For Mary, on the other hand, feeling rejected with a decent amount of "I'm a failure" thrown in, caused her to develop an "I'll show you" attitude, meaning she was determined to create an extraordinary life to show her mother that she was successful and therefore loveable. This not only influenced the development of her likeable personality, but also made her financially successful, enabling her to give back to those in need in enormous ways. So her meanings fostered a lot of good.

But there often comes a point when the meanings we've created no longer serve us. For example, if you are always pleasing people— so you feel like you never let them down, or disappoint them, so you can avoid feeling guilty—it is likely to become exhausting after a while and could deplete your adrenal glands, and this may be the basis of your health problems. Mary ate huge volumes of food most nights as a way of avoiding the reality that all she ever really wanted was her mother's love. She would never have seen that because the hatred she'd constructed was so vast. When Mary could see that her mother had actually always loved her, her food patterns and body fat changed significantly.

Sometimes all it takes is a glimpse of the "truth" for a shift to occur, leading to an effortless change in food behavior and a gentle letting-go of the blanket of protection (body fat) that may have been carried for decades. For others, I take them through a process that I created many years ago to help people better obtain the health outcomes they were seeking. I was first exposed to the concept of subconscious rules in a book called *Awaken the Giant Within* by Tony Robbins. I recognize the significant contribution Tony has made to this world by deciphering so much of human psychology, and for his insights and strategies.

What are your rules?

The process I guide people through at my weekend events involves first recognizing and writing down what currently has to happen for them to feel love. Then I ask them to write down what currently has to happen for them to feel rejected.

Question: *What emotion do you want to feel regularly?*

Answer: *Love*

Write down what currently has to happen for you to feel love.

When I do this exercise with female love bugs, common responses often include:

- *He has to look at me with soft, gentle eyes, smile like he really means it, and reach out and touch my hand all at the same time.*

- *He can never raise his voice at me.*

- *He can never use anything but a nice tone with me.*

- *He can never be late.*

- *He can never play computer games when there are jobs to do around the house.*

- *He always has to notice when I am overwhelmed and help me, even if I haven't asked.*

- *No one can ever ignore me!*

So you may find when you review your answers that you start giggling or get teary, as you begin to see the conflicts. Doing this exercise for the first time may also make you realize how tough you're making it for yourself to feel and experience a given emotion, in this case love. Notice if your language is absolute, featuring words such as "never" and "always," so your nervous system can only feel love when *all* of these things are happening at the same time.

Additionally, most people have no idea what they really want, so how on earth is anyone else supposed to? No wonder people get so angry with their partners and don't understand what's really behind it. They never feel loved because their partner doesn't do *all* of the above! Besides, how do you explain to someone that they "can *never* use anything but a nice tone" with you? For one thing, the way one person defines a "nice" tone will be entirely different from someone else. We are very funny, we humans.

Rejection list

The next step is to create your current rejection list.

Question: *What emotion is really painful for you to feel?*

Answer: *Rejection*

Write down what currently has to happen for you to feel rejected. For example:

- *If my partner raises his/her voice at me.*

- *If my partner doesn't look me in the eye.*

- *If a colleague, who usually stops by to say hi when they walk past my office, doesn't.*

- *If someone ignores me.*

- *If someone questions my work and asks me why I've done what I've done.*

• • • • • • • • • • • • • • • • • •

A "rejection" story that exemplifies what I mean involved a client and one of her colleagues. My client didn't enjoy her job, so the highlight of her day was her colleague stopping by her office to chat on his way back from the coffee machine. They mostly chatted about things other than work and he stopped by every day. Until he didn't.

One day, he walked past (she said "marched past") and didn't stop to chat. In that moment, many females would react internally in the same way my client did and ask, "What have I done?" It can take us two minutes, two days, two weeks, or two years before we pause to think, "I wonder what might be going on for him." By then, you have tortured yourself with every possible scenario of how you could have offended him, even though you hadn't had an interaction with him since your chat the day before.

Perhaps he just had piles of work to get through and he forgot to stop. Maybe he had a sick child and was racing back to his desk in case the phone rang. I could hypothesize for hours. My point is, save yourself a whole lot of heartache, rejection, exhaustion, distraction, mean self-talk and "unresourceful" eating or excessive drinking, and ask yourself, "I wonder what might be going on for him (or her)." He might appreciate your concern. And on the off chance he is upset with you, you can sort it out immediately.

You can see that the items on the list of rejection scenarios above could easily happen 50 times a day. How many times do you think this particular woman experienced "rejection" in a day compared to "love" based on these two sets of "rules"? Even though you don't walk around all day saying, "I feel rejected, I feel rejected, I feel rejected," you might still feel flat, lousy, depressed, angry, irritated, and frustrated. You may loathe yourself because you have scratched your "rejection" itch 50 times that day, and your perception is that you touched on love only twice.

Let me remind you again, *none* of this is conscious. *None* of these thoughts are cognitive in nature. They reveal themselves in your body as a momentary sick feeling in your tummy or a momentary spasm in your back, for example. In that moment, if you wanted to, you could access your sense of rejection. But you've conditioned your conscious mind never to go there (unless it is glaringly obvious). How often you subconsciously "feel" rejection and how often you subconsciously "feel" love is the fuel for your life. Your fuel, your juice, your passion won't show up if you are spending most of your day touching on rejection and feeling like you aren't enough. And it is at the end of a day like this, that, if food is your "comfort," your "drug," the way you "bolt," then no amount of "willpower" will ever be able to override your subconscious desperation to avoid actually *feeling* the rejection that, when you were a small child, your conscious mind perceived but decided was just too painful to feel.

There are numerous ways to get out of dodge, to alter the above scenario and patterns. The first involves rewriting your rules about what has to happen for you to feel love and rejection and, with practice, your emotional landscape will begin to change. After all, the first set of rules went in without you being conscious of it. Now it's time to direct your own rules and choose ones that actually serve you! It is, however, essential to practice saying your new rules once you have them. They can be great to recite while out for a walk. People driving by won't notice or if they do, they will just think you are singing (if you are concerned).

Rewrite your own rules

Playfully approach rewriting the rules for any of your emotions. The whole idea is to make the emotions you want to feel, in this case love, or success, for example, really easy to feel, and, with the new rules we write, to make it really difficult to feel the emotions that debilitate us such as rejection or failure.

Write new rules for yourself about how you will feel your desired emotion, or what I call your "green" emotion, for example love. Make it really easy to feel! It is vital you keep the green emotion in your control, not reliant on anyone else.

Start the spiel with "Anytime I…" and write "or" in between each rule.

For example, "Anytime I…

- *Smile or*

- *Appreciate nature or*

- *Eat food that nourishes me or*

- *Drink a glass of water or*

- *Hear birdsong or*

- *Exercise or*

- *Write in my diary* or

- *Read a book* or

- *Light a candle* or

- *Laugh* or...

I feel love."

Read these out loud every day for a month and move your body as you say them. You might sway gently, dance, walk, or use powerful arm actions. Pay attention when you smile and, after a while, notice a different level of happiness start to emerge from a feeling inside. You will hear more birdsong. You will drink more water, and each time you will not just be listening and appreciating and quenching your thirst, but your nervous system will start to feel "love" from the activities you do that, for you, now demonstrate love toward yourself.

Now write a new rule for yourself about how you will feel your "red" emotion, for example rejection. Make it really hard to feel. Make it about you rather than anyone else. Start with "Only if I were consistently to indulge in the debilitating, unresourceful emotion of... [for example rejection] instead of remembering that..."

... only I determine how I feel and respond to others, and I have not walked in anyone else's shoes.

It is so important to read your new rules aloud and combine them with motion. This helps engage your nervous system, allowing your subconscious to be reeducated with rules and meanings that will serve you and allow you to feel and acknowledge how truly amazing you are.

• • • • • • • • • • • • • • • • • • •

Network spinal analysis (NSA) and Somato respiratory integration (SRI)

A second modality I want to share with you is called Network Spinal Analysis (NSA), a powerful, non-cracking form of chiropractic that also encompasses a particular type of breathing called Somato (body) Respiratory Integration (SRI). It is truly a phenomenal practice. We'll be looking at a third way to alter your subconscious responses by applying a spectacular and gentle process called the Emotional Matrix ("Em–Matrix").

There is a school of thought that our body carries memories of what we have experienced in life. You may have noticed a person's posture perhaps, and used language to describe them (for example) as "having the weight of the world on their shoulders." Often, based on their perception of their own life, people will indeed feel this way. An NSA practitioner believes that, via your nervous system, your body stores experiences, both physical and emotional, and that our postures, even subtle ones, hold us in these patterns of belief. An NSA practitioner sees many different defense postures in a day's work and gently helps the body begin to shift into more resourceful postures. What is a great gift, is that as the body changes, so do the physical and emotional resources available to that person. And that can help change the choices they make.

When you think about your spine being the "connector" between your brain and your organs, you begin to get an idea of why your spine's health is worth optimizing... for it offers you a gateway between your body and your mind.

Developed by an incredibly gifted man, Donny Epstein, NSA involves gentle, precise touch to the spine that cues the brain to create new wellness strategies. Through working on the physical structure of the body, behavioral change unfolds literally effortlessly. Through SRI, people are educated to the body's rhythms and their own inner wisdom using focused attention, gentle breath, movement and touch. A big part of SRI behind the scenes is helping the nervous system feel "safe", a place from which new perceptions, healing and optimal health can transform. I personally love these approaches to health and as with many modalities, they really need to be experienced to be "understood."

The Em-Matrix

What if I told you that every single emotion is here to serve you? What if I told you that every emotion has a gift for you? What if I told you that every emotion has a message for you and that once you hear it, a space will remain for your truth, your core essence to expand into? And what if I told you that instead of delving back into your past to help you cognitively understand why you eat "unresourcefully," we could instead simply and gently explore the emotions and the patterns that exist today. Welcome to the Em-Matrix, a concept and a process the world so desperately needs. Open your mind and heart to this.

An incredibly gifted and generous woman called Deborah Battersby is the founder of a concept called Em-Matrix. Having studied with Deb, I've discovered how powerful her work is in the way it allows people gently to see how every emotion that we may perceive to be negative, has actually come to serve us. Deb has created a process that you can be guided through (or with a little experience, you can take yourself through) and that will allow what I've been referring to as your subconscious mind to communicate the real reason a particular pattern or emotion keeps showing up in your life.

For example, you really want to quit your job and start your own business, but, every time you come close, you feel frightened. Fear can serve you or fear can hold you back. Guided by the fundamental principle of Em-Matrix that all emotion is here to serve, the gentle and effortless Em-Matrix process allows the "fear" to speak and communicate its wonderful intentions, which could include "to keep you safe" and "to offer wisdom." Yet fear may be holding you back from a life that somewhere in your heart could be enormously fulfilling. And when humans aren't fulfilled, many of them eat.

What I have now seen time and time again is that, once you see that a particular fear was there to help you and it had simply overstayed its welcome, you let it go and you allow your truth to fill the space where once the fear resided. The Em-Matrix process allows your subconscious to "speak" and as a result I've seen very anxious people go from being wired and highly stressed, to being calm and centered and mostly remain that way. This process positively impacts your nervous system because your old, subconscious thoughts and feelings that once silently wired and unwittingly consumed you now give you strength, passion, and insight.

A simple explanation of how this happens is that when you have a perception that an emotion you feel is negative, your SNS activates; the "fight-or-flight" response. It does this partly because, in that moment, you judge yourself. And if you continue to touch on this emotion frequently and subsequently have too much time with the SNS activated, it will bring with it all of the consequences of too many stress hormones, including cortisol. If this pattern or this emotion stops you from truly resting, your PNS is unable to do the rest and repair work it needs to, which, as you now know, drives its own set of consequences.

When it comes to emotions, it can be the emotions that we literally keep "stuffed" inside ourselves that may drive us to indulge in addictions to keep us distracted from the emotional pain. That's the flight. That's the bolting and the getting out of dodge. The never wanting to return "home" to yourself because you perceive it is too painful and, gosh, also because that big scary piece of pain that you were so clever to stuff back down inside yourself with the cake you ate after dinner might bubble to the surface. So you keep bolting and never *feeling* what it really is that's present. The fight, on the other hand, is either "suppressed" or it "explodes" in angry outbursts or rage, and the consequences of that not only affect the individual exploding but usually the people around them, too. Whatever you then say to yourself (a story) about who you must be to explode like that is powerful and keeps your SNS dominant with everything that it creates.

The Em-Matrix is a wonderful process to experience. It is such a spectacular yet gentle way to change the patterns and emotional landscape of your life. The distinctions, transformations, and breakthroughs it offers have the potential to change that landscape—to change the world really. Imagine how much less cortisol we would all make!

Signs your emotional landscape needs some support

- You are human ☺ (i.e., most people need to explore this area of their lives)

- You eat emotionally

- You have good nutrition and health knowledge, but this doesn't translate consistently into good health and nutrition choices

- You don't understand why you do what you do when you know what you know.

EMOTIONS SOLUTIONS

I hope you now see how your thoughts and beliefs are just as powerful, if not more powerful, than anything you put in your mouth, and so taking the time to understand your emotions is a vital piece of your weight-loss puzzle. The following solutions are all about helping you to do just that.

- Eating in a way that doesn't serve you is a way you distance yourself from how things are when they are not how you want them to be. Ask yourself what you want to distance yourself from—the state of your marriage, the way your children speak to you, the hurt from your father sending you to boarding school at a young age—and really experience the fact that how you eat will not change these things. You need other strategies, not lousy eating, to transform that pain. It is never about the food.

- Do the "Food is…" exercise (*see page 181*) and learn what role you are really asking food to play in your life. Once you see that it is more joy or more fun or comfort you are seeking, you can schedule ways to experience these emotions through means that don't take away from your health.

- Explore your subconscious rules about what has to happen for you to feel the emotions you want to feel, as well as those you seek to avoid, using the strategy outlined. It can offer powerful insights into why you may find changing food behaviors so challenging (if you do) and you will be able to bring much more compassion to yourself with the new understanding you gain. Rewrite your rules!

- Bodywork and/or breathing processes may assist such as NSA and SRI. Seek out skilled practitioners to support you with this if it appeals.

- Remember that every emotion is here to serve you; some just overstay their welcome. If there is a recurring emotional pattern in your life, identify it, for example anger and then say to the anger—"If it is true that you are here to serve me, what is it that you are here to do?" In every moment we are responding from love or fear. There is no in between. And quite often when there is an emotion that has overstayed its welcome, it originally appeared to help or protect you. But now it may be destructive, to you or others. Processes such as Em-Matrix, help you get to the heart of what the emotional pattern is really all about.

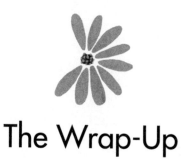

The Wrap-Up

After all of this talk about food, hormones, alcohol, coffee, and body size, I want to remind you that it is never about the food. Nor is it about the hormones, and yet, at the same time, it is about them because you will feel so much better if you address, for example, your estrogen dominance or insulin resistance. But hear this, please hear this... you would never want the garbage or the harmful amounts you swallow, if you knew who you really are. If you truly had a deep appreciation of how magnificent you are or saw the light that shines inside you, regardless of how dim you tell yourself you are or how dim you think you need to be to fit in, you would never treat yourself that way. And when you decide you don't want the rubbish—rather than you going without the garbage because someone told you to—everything changes, including the estrogen dominance, the insulin resistance, and the body fat you no longer need. You feel safe because you have *you*.

But in this space you are not even focused on your size. You *know* you are a remarkable human, and you have such a deep appreciation and level of care for yourself that an excess of anything no longer appeals or even appears in your life. When we choose to drink alcohol, we are spitting in the eye of our greatness, dulling ourselves so we feel less, do less, shine less. Sharing a drink over a celebration is a very different scenario from the daily grind of alcohol, and the sharing is to be enjoyed if you like to do so. Of course alcohol can be good for your soul. And only you know whether you are nourishing your soul or dimming your light.

You shut down your insight, you shut down your feelings, and you shut down your truth when you rely on alcohol to "relax" in the evenings. What you are actually saying when you drink alcohol in excess is that you can't face your reality. Perhaps you can't face it that you can't bear another moment of baby talk (even though you love your children very much), and that feeling leads you to believe that you are a bad person. So, you drink to "cope" with the crazy 5 to 6 p.m. period. Or because you had an affair and, even though you stayed in your original relationship, you are bored with your life. You drink to make the life you chose more bearable. Maybe your daily alcohol intake began when you started a new job, one you didn't really want. And you can't face it that you feel so resentful toward your husband, with whom you once shared a beautiful, intimate marriage, because he bought a business that did not do well financially, forcing you back to work against your will. So you drink each evening with a bitter taste in your mouth, justifying your consumption through your story that you deserve it because you work so bleeping hard. What you actually deserve is to see your own brilliance and then live from that place. You would never want to shut off from that, and alcohol abuse effortlessly exits your life.

Knowing this does not mean that you now have permission to judge yourself every time you want to drink alcohol. If you drink it, enjoy it. I'm not telling you what to do or what not to do. I simply want you to see why you do what you do, especially if what you do is harming you.

If you truly want amazing health that feels effortless, then begin to observe your own behaviors. For example, when you want the alcohol or the food that doesn't serve you (for any of the above alcohol-based examples can be replaced with food patterns that don't serve you), ask yourself what you really want. It might be rest, a hug, or appreciation for all you do in a day, or it may be to forget the pain in your heart because someone you love is very ill. All of these things are just pain, emotional pain. And emotional pain will not kill you. In fact, I've learned that quite often it can offer the most magical insight into a part of you that is precious and powerful all at once... often precisely what you are searching for in the food. Imagine realizing that the precious and powerful piece inside you is the most extraordinary best friend you could ever ask to walk beside you through life.

My intention for this book was to show you through science and emotion, and the links between them, that it is always about more than the food. Food is simply a way that we cope. Weight, whether it is too much or too little, is a by-product of your coping strategies and a reflection of your beliefs. Excess weight is what happens when you use food to flatten your life.

From this moment on I want you to spend at least five minutes every day recognizing all that you contribute to this world, just by being who you are. And let that recognition light a flame inside you that with every day grows stronger and brighter from the kindness you show yourself through your lifestyle choices and your thoughts. And may that light guide you home to the magnificence you have always been.

• • • • • • • • • • • • •

References and Resources

My website, www.drlibby.com, offers free information and recipes as well as information about my events, books and online courses. The events and educational tools are designed to take you further in your *Accidentally Overweight* journey if you feel you want more in the way of dietary, hormonal and emotional guidance and support. I speak all over the world and announce where I'm going to be presenting in my monthly newsletter. Be sure to pop your email address in the form on the website and I look forward to meeting you in person soon.

I have included this section for numerous purposes. First, if you enjoy science there are some fascinating scientific publications listed here. These are written in a scientific reference format. There are also books I've referenced in the text, listed in full in this section if further reading in a particular area interests you. Finally, the purpose of this section is to offer you additional resources, which include techniques you may wish to explore to help you understand your emotional landscape better.

Not all of the puzzle pieces have additional resources listed as I have studied and read widely (sometimes from very geeky biochemistry textbooks) and this book is the culmination of my knowledge, experience, observation and intuition to date.

References

1. Horvath, K. and Perman, J. "Autistic disorder and gastrointestinal disease," *Current Opinions in Pediatrics*, 2002; 14 (5): 583–7

2. Horvath, K. and Perman, J. "Autism and gastrointestinal symptoms," *Current Gastroenterology Reports*, 2002; 4(3): 251–8

3. Horvath, K. Papadimitriou, J. Rabsztyn, A. Drachenberg. C. Tildon, J. "Gastrointestinal abnormalities in children with autistic disorders," *Journal of Pediatrics*, 1999; 135(5): 559–63

4. Jin, W. Wang, H. Ji, Y. Hu, Q. Yan, W. Chen, G. Yin, H. "Increased intestinal inflammatory response and gut barrier dysfunction in Nrf2-deficient mice after traumatic brain injury," *Cytokine*, 2008; 44(1): 135–40

5. Cade, R. Privette, M. Fregly, M. Rowland, N. Sun, Z. Zele, V. Wagemaker, H. Edelstein, C. "Autism and schizophrenia: Intestinal disorders," *Nutritional Neuroscience*, 2000; 3(1): 57–72

6. Rock, C. Natarajan, L. Pu, M.Thomson, C. Flatt, S. Caan, B. Gold, E. Al-Delaimy, W. Newman, V. Hajek, R. Stefanick, M. Pierce, J. "Longitudinal biological exposure to carotenoids is associated with breast cancer-free survival in the women's healthy eating and living study," *Cancer Epidemiology, Biomarkers & Prevention*, 2009; 18(2), 486–94

7. Arcidiacono, B. Iiritano, S. Nocera, A. Possidente, K. Nevolo, M. Ventura, V. Foti, D. Chiefari, E. Brunetti, A. "Insulin resistance and cancer risk: An overview of the pathogenetic mechanisms," *Experimental Diabetes Research*, 2012; Article ID 789174: 12 pages

8. Aceves, C. Anguiano, B. Delgado, G. "Is iodine a gatekeeper of the integrity of the mammary gland?" *Journal of Mammary Gland Biology and Neoplasia*, 2005; 10(2): 189–96

9. Stoddard, F. Brooks, A. Eskin, B. Johannes, G. "Iodine alters gene expression in the MCF7 breast cancer cell line: evidence for an anti-estrogen effect of iodine," *International journal of medical sciences*, 2008; 5(4): 189–96

10. Venturi, S. "Is there a role for iodine in breast diseases?" *The Breast*, 2001; 10(5): 379–82

11. Ley, R. Turnbaugh, P. Klein, S. Gordon, J. "Microbial ecology: Human gut microbes associated with obesity," *Nature*, 2006; 444(7122): 1022–23

12. Lustig, R. "Childhood obesity: behavioral aberration or biochemical drive? Reinterpreting the first law of thermodynamics," *Nature Clinical Practice, Endocrinology & Metabolism Review*, 2006; 2 (8): 447–57

13. Heymsfield, S. Greenberg, A. Fujioka, K. Dixon, R. Kushner, R. Hunt, T. Lubina, J. Patane, J. Self, B. Hunt, P. McCamish, M. "Recombinant leptin for weight loss in obese and lean adults: a randomized, controlled, dose-escalation trial," *Journal of the American Medical Association*, 1999; 282: 1568–75

14. Jenkins, D. Wolever, T. Taylor, R. Barker, H. Fielden, H. Baldwin, J. Bowling, A. Newman, H. Jenkins, A. Goff, D. "Glycemic index of foods: a physiological basis for carbohydrate exchange," *American Journal of Clinical Nutrition*, 1981; 34(3): 362–6

Resources

Digestion

Cade, R. Privette, M. Fregly, M. Rowland, N. Sun, Z. Zele, V. Wagemaker, H, Edelstein, C. "Autism and schizophrenia: Intestinal disorders." *Nutritional Neuroscience*, 2000; 3(1): 57–72

Horvath, K. and Perman, J. "Autistic disorder and gastrointestinal disease," *Current Opinions in Pediatrics*, 2002; 14(5): 583–7

Horvath, K. and Perman, J. "Autism and gastrointestinal symptoms," *Current Gastroenterology Reports*, 2002; 4(3): 251–8

Horvath, K. Papadimitriou, J. Rabsztyn, A. Drachenberg. C. Tildon. J.T. "Gastrointestinal abnormalities in children with autistic disorders," *Journal of Pediatrics*, 1999; 135(5): 559–63

Jin, W. Wang, H. Ji, Y. Hu, Q. Yan, W. Chen, G. Yin, H. "Increased intestinal inflammatory response and gut barrier dysfunction in Nrf2-deficient mice after traumatic brain injury," *Cytokine*, 2008; 44(1): 135–40

Sex Hormones

Aceves, C. Anguiano, B. Delgado, G. "Is iodine a gatekeeper of the integrity of the mammary gland?" *Journal of Mammary Gland Biology and Neoplasia*, 2005; 10(2): 189–96

Arcidiacono, B. Iiritano, S. Nocera, A. Possidente, K. Nevolo, M. Ventura, V. Foti, D. Chiefari, E. Brunetti, A. "Insulin resistance and cancer risk: An overview of the pathogenetic mechanisms," *Experimental Diabetes Research*, 2012; Article ID 789174, 12 pages

Naish, F. and Roberts, J. *Better Health for Better Babies* series (Sydney: Random House, 1997)

Northrup, C. *Women's Bodies, Women's Wisdom* (London: Judy Piatkus Ltd, 1998)

Rock, C. Natarajan, L. Pu, M. Thomson, C. Flatt, S. Caan, B. Gold, E. Al-Delaimy, W. Newman, V. Hajek, R. Stefanick, M. Pierce, J. "Longitudinal biological exposure to carotenoids is associated with breast cancer-free survival in the women's healthy eating and living study." *Cancer Epidemiology, Biomarkers & Prevention*, 2009; 18(2): 486–94

Stoddard, F. Brooks, A. Eskin, B. Johannes, G. "Iodine alters gene expression in the MCF7 breast cancer cell line: evidence for an anti-estrogen effect of iodine," *International journal of medical sciences*, 2008; 5(4): 189–96

Venturi, S. "Is there a role for iodine in breast diseases?" *The Breast*, 2001; 10(5): 379–82

Gut Bacteria

Gottschall, E. *Breaking the Vicious Cycle* (Baltimore: Kirkton Press Ltd, 1994; for the Specific Carbohydrate Diet)

Ley, R. Turnbaugh, P. Klein, S. Gordon, J. "Microbial ecology: Human gut microbes associated with obesity," *Nature*, 2006; 444(7122): 1022–23

The Thyroid

Coates, K. and Perry, V. *Embracing the Warrior: An Essential Guide for Women* (Burleigh Heads, Arteriol Press, 2007)

Hay, L. *You Can Heal Your Life* (Carlsbad: Hay House Inc, 2004)

Insulin

Chek, P. *How to Eat, Move and Be Healthy!* (Encinitas: C.H.E.K Institute LLC, 2004)

Heymsfield, S. Greenberg, A. Fujioka, K. Dixon, R. Kushner, R. Hunt, T. Lubina, J. Patane, J. Self, B. Hunt, P. McCamish, M. "Recombinant leptin for weight loss in obese and lean adults: a randomized, controlled, dose-escalation trial," *Journal of the American Medical Association*, 1999; 282: 1568–75

Isganaitis, E. and Lustig, R. "Fast food, central nervous system insulin resistance, and obesity," *Arteriosclerosis Thrombosis Vascular Biology*, 2005; 25: 2451–62

Lustig, R. "Childhood obesity: behavioral aberration or biochemical drive? Reinterpreting the first law of thermodynamics," *Nature Clinical Practice, Endocrinology & Metabolism* Review, 2006; 2(8): 447–57

Lustig, R. "The 'skinny' on childhood obesity: How our Western environment starves kids' brains," *Pediatric Annals*, 2006; 35(12): 899–907

Emotions

Epstein, D. *The 12 Stages of Healing* (San Rafael: Amber-Allen Publishers, 1994)

Hay, L. *You Can Heal Your Life* (Carlsbad: Hay House Inc, 2004)

Robbins, A. *Awaken the Giant Within* (London: Simon & Schuster Ltd, 1992)

● ● ● ● ● ● ● ● ● ● ● ●

Index

Page references in *italic* represent figures and tables.

ABOUT THE AUTHOR

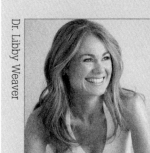

Dr. Libby Weaver

Dr. Libby Weaver (PhD) is a leading nutritional biochemist, an eight-time #1 best-selling author and an international speaker.

Dr. Libby graduated from the University of Newcastle in Australia with a Bachelor of Health Science Nutrition and Dietetics with Honors, and a PhD in Biochemistry. She combines this knowledge with two decades of clinical practice working with patients from all walks of life, from stay-at-home mums to Hollywood stars.

When addressing any health concern, Dr. Libby's three-pillar approach examines the biochemical, nutritional and emotional reasons behind what might be driving the body to behave in a certain way. As an internationally respected writer and speaker Dr. Libby has shared the stage with Tony Robbins, Dr. Oz, Sir Richard Branson and Marianne Williamson. She has also spoken at TEDx as well as frequently hosting her own events.

Dr. Libby runs a successful Holistic Nutrition Consultancy, which provides people all over the world with nutritional consultations and empowering seminars and retreats. She has been featured in numerous media publications including *The Times*, *The Huffington Post*, *Sydney Morning Herald*, and the *Australian Women's Weekly*, and she appears regularly on breakfast television.

Armed with an abundance of knowledge, scientific research and a true desire to help others see their own light and magnificence, Dr. Libby empowers and inspires people to take charge of their health and happiness.

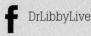 DrLibbyLive   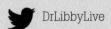 DrLibbyLive   drlibby

www.drlibby.com

229

We hope you enjoyed this Hay House book. If you'd like to receive our online catalog featuring additional information on Hay House books and products, or if you'd like to find out more about the
Hay Foundation, please contact:

Hay House, Inc., P.O. Box 5100, Carlsbad, CA 92018-5100
(760) 431-7695 or (800) 654-5126
(760) 431-6948 (fax) or (800) 650-5115 (fax)
www.hayhouse.com® • www.hayfoundation.org

• • • • • • • • • • • • • •

Published and distributed in Australia by: Hay House Australia Pty. Ltd.,
18/36 Ralph St., Alexandria NSW 2015
Phone: 612-9669-4299 • *Fax:* 612-9669-4144 • www.hayhouse.com.au

Published and distributed in the United Kingdom by: Hay House UK, Ltd.,
Astley House, 33 Notting Hill Gate, London W11 3JQ
Phone: 44-20-3675-2450 • *Fax:* 44-20-3675-2451 • www.hayhouse.co.uk

Published and distributed in the Republic of South Africa by:
Hay House SA (Pty), Ltd., P.O. Box 990, Witkoppen 2068
info@hayhouse.co.za • www.hayhouse.co.za

Published in India by: Hay House Publishers India,
Muskaan Complex, Plot No. 3, B-2, Vasant Kunj, New Delhi 110 070
Phone: 91-11-4176-1620 • *Fax:* 91-11-4176-1630 • www.hayhouse.co.in

Distributed in Canada by: Raincoast Books,
2440 Viking Way, Richmond, B.C. V6V 1N2
Phone: 1-800-663-5714 • *Fax:* 1-800-565-3770 • www.raincoast.com

• • • • • • • • • • • • • •

Take Your Soul on a Vacation

Visit www.HealYourLife.com® to regroup,
recharge, and reconnect with your own magnificence.
Featuring blogs, mind-body-spirit news, and
life-changing wisdom from Louise Hay and friends.

Visit www.HealYourLife.com today!